No Ordinary Woman
Tips for conscious, creative, and healthy living

Gabrielle Javier-Cerulli, MA

We, women, are incredible beings. We juggle so many roles these days. With so many demands on our time from work, family, school, and friends we sometimes miss information that can better our lives. The purpose of this publication is to help you explore new ideas and, ultimately, to be entertaining. It's like a research paper covering all of which I'm passionate.

This publication is protected under the US Copyright Act of 1976 and all other applicable international, federal, state, and local laws, and all rights are reserved.

Please do not reprint any part of it without written consent from the author, Gabrielle Javier-Cerulli, except for the inclusion of brief quotations in a review. If you do use a brief quotation or reference this publication in any way, please link to www.TheExpressiveArtsCoach.com.

Please note that much of this book is based on personal and research experience. Although Gabrielle Javier-Cerulli has made attempts to achieve accuracy of the content, she assumes no responsibility for errors or omissions.

Use this information as you see fit, and at your own risk. Please use your own judgment. Nothing in this book should replace common sense, legal, medical, financial, or other professional advice. This book is meant to share information and entertain the reader.

Enjoy!

Cover Image by Erik Reis of Portugal
One day I looked at over 3,000 images for this book. When I saw Erik's photo, I knew it was *the* one! His work can be seen at www.erikreis.com

DEDICATION

This book is dedicated to my mother, Mary Ann
who is no ordinary woman
and
to all extra-ordinary women (like you reading this book!)

CONTENTS

ACKNOWLEDGMENTS

My heart is full with all the people I wish to thank. At the top of the list are the two dudes in my life.

First a special loving thanks to my husband, Anthony for his support in this and all my endeavors.

To my son, whose joyful presence keeps me smiling.

To my sister Renae for being no ordinary woman and guiding her little sister throughout life.

To my brother Rafael for being a role model of entrepreneurial dedication and success.

To my niece Rachel for being no ordinary woman and someone with whom I can discuss the mysteries of life.

To my younger niece and nephews, Ellen, Patrick and Croix for providing endless hours of entertainment. It's a joy to watch you all grow.

To Lori for being no ordinary woman and being my Friend.

To Reid and Jen for your loving friendship for over two decades.

To all my amazing friends, many thanks for always being there. I want to hang out with you all more often.

To anyone who is reading this, I deeply appreciate you for taking the time to read my first published book.

Conscious Living

What does *conscious living* mean to you? I asked a friend not too long ago and she thought about it for a moment and said it reminds her of yoga. Another friend admitted it sounds pretty mystical. While conscious living may include taking care of your body, it isn't limited to yoga and it certainly isn't mystical. It's about everyday living with awareness.

My personal definition of conscious living means to be fully awake and aware of how I am living, how I move through life, and trying my best **not to live on autopilot**. Lifestyle patterns handed down by previous generations are questioned because there's a determination that better alternatives exist. I'm also conscientious of how my actions affect broader systems such as my family, community, environment, and society at large. I believe I'm responsible for my life and happiness and since this is my one precious life, I should give it my all. I choose not to live saddled with negativity and it's a continuous process to let go of old programming and past wounds. For anyone trying to live consciously, there's a heightened sensitivity to well...everything. There's concern for other people, for nature, for animals, for skin care products, for the air, for water, for positive energy, for children, and the list goes on.

Of course, I'm not in this state every single day but for the majority of the time I am. Would life be easier not thinking about *stuff*? It probably would be. *Ignorance is bliss*, you know. But all this *stuff* is important to me.

We all know Socrates's words of wisdom, "The unexamined life is not worth living." But do we all take heed of these words? Are you fully present in your life? Without knowing your depths, you will not be truly aware of your possibilities. Now is the time to dive deeply into the pool of self-discovery!

In Chapter 1 Know Thyself, I'll discuss eight different ways you can get to know yourself on a deeper level. Chapter 2 Finding Your Life's Purpose, reviews how you can find your true purpose so you can have a phenomenal life. Chapter 3 Being a Mama, is a hodgepodge of ideas geared towards conscious parenting. Chapter 4 Your Moolah, outlines how you can have a better relationship with something so vital in your life...your money. I hope you learn some new stuff here and apply it to your life. You may experience a positive shift.

CHAPTER 1

KNOW THYSELF

Are you a Beggar, Wounded Healer, or Goddess?
Know Your Archetypes.

Familiar personality types and recurring human energy patterns can be found worldwide. During my travels I noticed how similar people are. No matter if you go to the island of Cebu, Philippines, ride a rickshaw in Trivandrum India, wander around the streets of London's Covent Garden, or hang out in the bars of Fells Point in Baltimore, Maryland there seem to be certain types of people. There are the loyal nationalists who believe their country is number one; the artists and creative types who are making art, music, dancing, producing handicrafts, and performing in theaters; the intelligentsia and the academics who are serious about their chosen field; the sports fanatics, the hustlers, the blowhards, the princesses, the politicians; and so on. The different essences of a person holds a recurring energy and that's what an archetype is.

Movies and television shows frequently feature an archetype such as the Hero, the Damsel, the Tramp, the Athlete, the Hedonist, and Computer/Technology Geek.

What are your recurring energy patterns? Who are your archetypes and how can they help you navigate through life? According to Carolyn Myss of www.myss.com, we all have twelve archetypes that are influential to us. Of the twelve, four archetypes are the same for everyone. Those four are: Child, Victim, Saboteur, and Prostitute (not as in a sex worker but instead reflecting on what of ourselves we are giving away for material gain).   The other eight archetypes are personal guiding archetypes. During an archetype reading you'll discover your other eight archetypes. Readings can be done on your own or with a trained reader.

After working on my own for a bit using Myss' website as a guide, I decided to work with a professional since I was faced with a life changing decision about my career. There's a listing of trained archetype readers by state and country on Myss' website. I found Ellen Rusling listed under "archetype readings." She looked like a Sage and Wise Woman (two more archetypes). Although archetype readings can be done on your own, like anything, having a professional guide will deepen your self-discovery experience. A trained professional will take you places you can't go on your own. There's a great need for objective input, which must come from someone other than yourself.

With Ellen's help, I uncovered my other eight archetypes and learned how they assist in distinct areas of my life. A few of my archetypes are Networker, Leader, and Artist/Creative. Becoming aware of and fully embracing of all my archetypes, but especially these three, made the big career decision easier. The decision was made with confidence since I fully knew who I was and what I bring/offer to the outside world. What would your archetypes be? Wounded Healer? Mother? Innovator? Warrior? Beggar? Once you know you can claim your roles in life with steadfastness and joy. This knowledge can help you decide on careers, help with your marketing message, and help with relationships. Think about this example...if you're a Goddess who embodies the Divine Feminine, but you're trying to market your graphics arts business as mundane and corporate, then your business will probably suffer because your true voice and self aren't shining through. It may behoove you to infuse your femininity into your work and reach out to others who will appreciate your unique approach.

Look to the Stars for Answers?

As a kid my Mom bought those little rolled up weekly astrology readings. I vividly remember playing with the little plastic tubes and unrolling the scrolls which revealed interesting images of Virgo, Taurus, the planets and stars. So astrology, looking to the stars and planets for guidance, was instilled in me from a very early age. Mom also had dream books around and received an occasional card reading using playing cards instead of the traditional tarot cards with cups, swords, wands, and coins. However, she never took the metaphysical information too seriously. It was more of a curiosity she wanted satisfy. Consequently, I dabbled with astrology but never took it seriously as well.

However, a couple years ago a woman contacted me about her journey into expressive arts facilitation since we're in the same field.[1] She shared how she had relocated to San Luis Obispo, California because of her astrocartology reading, and now her professional and personal lives are thriving. Astrocartology is another name for relocation astrology. I'd heard of relocation astrology before but this woman's inspiring story piqued my interest. If I could figure out *where* I belong, maybe all the rest would fall into place. At the time of this printing I've lived in eleven states in the United States and four countries overseas. So, I often get asked, "Where would you *really* like to live?" I translate this question as: Where would I like to grow roots and stay until I die? So far, I can't answer that. There are positives and negatives to all of the places I've been. But now that I have child, *maybe* it is time to find *the* place to finally call home. Could I finally have an answer to where I belong? I was interested in finding out.

During my astrocartology session with the relocation expert I

---

[1] If you're the woman from SLO, please send me an email at NOWnoordinarywoman@gmail.com. Your contact info was lost when switching computers.

shared my birthday date, time, and location. The entire world could have been reviewed but I opted for only USA to be reviewed. One day I'd like to hear what the rest of the world looks like for me. The premise for astrocartology is your astrological chart is projected to the Earth's surface. When a baby takes their first breath here on Earth the stars and planets were located at certain places in the sky. These celestial locations are then placed over a world map and this determines the reading. I was informed there are cities and states that would be good for my career but not so great for my relationships. There are a couple cities that would be great for getting things accomplished but not so good for my overall emotions. I think four sweet spots were found where career, health, and relationships were all positive. One is in another state only 4.5 hours away from where I'm currently living and the other is Miami, Florida. So...Miami I'm coming to visit one day!

I haven't made any major transitions or moves with this new information from the session. If I were single and didn't have any children it *might* be another story. Right now, this is just more information under my belt. It will not determine where I live or do business. Some people may take the information from their reading and change their lives by it. I choose to have it in my back pocket.

Also, if you are married and/or have children, it makes sense to do an astrocartology reading for each family member to see where the collective sweet spot would be.

After the relocation reading, I delved into learning about my birth chart. I suggest going in the reverse order. First learn about your birth chart. Then, if you feel you need more information, an astrocartology reading may be useful. Your birth chart reveals so much about you that it will enhance your relocation reading.

My birth chart revealed surprising truths. It includes information about my childhood, family members, mate, and passions. It also contains challenges I've encountered. Can all of this be a coincidence? I tend to think not. I learned to read my own birth chart by using www.astro.com. You simply input your birth time and location and it produces a birth chart for free. Even though I'm satisfied with what I found on my own, I do look forward to getting it done professionally by someone who has dedicated his or her life to this science. Birth charts are a thing of beauty. The circles, lines, patterns, and symbols are lovely. One area that stood out in my chart was Venus in my 10th house. The 10th house is the house of career and life purpose. Venus represents the arts, creativity, and beauty. So I'm in alignment with my path of being an artist, a writer, expressive arts coach, and the founder of the Global Network of Expressive Arts Facilitators. It's a nice feeling to get validation from the stars and planets!

Get Your Vision Board Created

At first glance a vision board looks like a collage poster that might hang on a teenager's bedroom wall. It's a bunch of magazine cutouts pasted to a big board. But this simple looking end-product is born from a deep and involved process. Helping people make a vision board is the most popular workshop that I offer. In order to give more people the opportunity to create their vision boards in the comfort of their home, I wrote an ebook, *Create Your Vision Board at Home: Learn How to Clarify Your Needs, Desires, and Goals Using Your Creativity,* which can be found at www.TheExpressiveArtsCoach.com/products. Every facilitator manages the vision board process differently. After years of client and workshop participant feedback, I now begin with a thorough self-reflection exercise. This warm-up exercise reviews 10 life areas by asking over 150 questions. Starting the process with this reflection time allows someone to make the most honest vision board. The life areas include: Home Environment, Personal Finances, Friendships, Primary Relationship, Family Relationships, Physical Health and Body Image, Fun and Leisure, Career/Life Purpose, Expressions of Creativity, and Spirituality. Humans are always looking to improve themselves and creating a vision board organizes your desires for you.

After answering the reflection questions, the next step is to find images to reflect the ways in which you want, need, and desire to shift your life. This is an enjoyable step because intuitive creativeness comes in. You get into a zone flipping through magazines or, if you're at a workshop, searching through piles and piles of precut images. It's always a joy to see how relaxed people get - their shoulders drop and they tend to breathe slowly and deeply. After completing the vision board, it's best to hang it in a location where you'll see it frequently. It doesn't need to be in your living room, but maybe behind the home office or bedroom door, next to a closet, under a bed (as long as you don't forget about it), or in the laundry room. Mine is currently on the wall behind the door in my home office. To see results, you'll want to review your board often, even daily, so the content sticks with you. Obviously everything on the board is not guaranteed but at least it's organized in one place. My clients have often update me on what has come to fruition for them. What would be on your board? Travel? Back to school? Lose weight? Better friendships?

Core Values

How do you know what you want in life if you aren't crystal clear about what you value? Doesn't everyone value the same thing? Nope. Some women value family more than others. For some women, adventure is a top priority, while for others a sense of security is of utmost importance.

Knowing your values clarifies why you do the things you do, why you get stressed out about certain things, and helps you make decisions. For instance, your neighbor just opened a cupcake bakery because her core values include adventure, risk-taking, creativity, and independence. You're envious because she's an entrepreneur, has a place in the community, laughs with the customers, and best of all, she's her own boss. But if having a secure, predictable lifestyle is at the top of your core values list and risk-taking is at the bottom, then this career choice wouldn't work for you because you'd be constantly stressed out. Remember that Cupcake Lady has to constantly hustle and her work is never finished. If the bakery alarm goes off at 4:00 am, she's the one that has to get up. If the bills are tight a particular month, she has to figure out how to eke out her payments. But her core values dictate that she is up for the challenge and feels more alive with this business venture.

How do you make a core values list? Simply write down 20 values that are important to you and then rate them from 1 to 20. Next, focus on the top 10 because these are your core values. This is the core of you – what is really important to you. This is a useful exercise to do with your partner, spouse, girlfriend or boyfriend, or even your business partner. Do both of you have similar outlooks on life? Doing this exercise together may help you answer why you can't see eye to eye and keep fighting. Or it might bring you closer together. I did this many years ago with my live-in boyfriend (now husband) and our top three core values were the same. Different order but the same. We did it again about ten years later, and again our top three values were the same. Do I hear a wave of people saying "awwww, ain't that sweet?" But you should know that beyond the top three, our values are very different! Knowing what he values puts things into perspective for me so I better understand him and us.

I just did the list again while writing this book and one of my three top ones have changed because I have child. So core values can change as your life changes.

Need help with your list? Check out the No Ordinary Woman Toolkit in the back of the book.

Gratitude Goes a Long Way

Be mindful of all the good in your life by writing a gratitude list on a daily or weekly basis. Writing or typing a list of people, objects, and opportunities you are thankful for reduces whining and melancholy. Really feel the positive energy in your body when doing this. It's a wonderful sensation. Consistent appreciation for your life promotes a sense of wellbeing and it will help you when times aren't so great. So when you're crying your eyes out on your bathroom floor because you lost someone you loved, or your job is awful, or your relationship isn't what you hoped, or for no reason at all, think back to your gratitude list to glean some hope and mollify your mood. Rereading your list during times like these can alleviate the pain just a bit.

It may be easiest to write three to five sentences each night before going to sleep. You can start your list with "I am so grateful for...." and just write what comes to mind. I tend to write on Sundays just before bed. In your gratitude journal you can list typical things like special people in your life, items that you use and adore, and new opportunities that came your way. I also include atypical things that I'm grateful for, such as indoor plumbing, affordable internet, the internet, Skype (being able to video visit with family and friends from around the world is awesome), and hiking trails I enjoy trekking with my family. Try writing new things each day. By not repeating yourself, your list will be fresh and your gratitude wide.

If you're more apt to do something on your computer instead of in a journal, then go to GratitudeLog[2]. It's tagline is "The Happiest Place on the Internet!" I just started on there and dig it so far but

---

[2] www.gratitudelog.com

not ready to give up my paper and pen just yet.

If you're a person who will never write a list, at least consider just naming what you're grateful for in your head. Next time at a red light or stuck in traffic or in a grocery check-out line, review all the good in your life. You can also do it while taking a shower, working out, falling asleep, waking up, or before a movie starts.

Inspiration File Folders

Does anyone else have stacks of articles, pictures, and handouts laying around on tables or the floor? There's value in these pages and can't be tossed out. Instead of being buried under all the useful words and cool images, collect them and put them in a folder or box to be read and viewed whenever you feel like it.

Keep one folder for images cut from magazines or greeting cards. Label it something interesting, like *My Inspirational Images, Images For Me ONLY*, or *Cool Things to Look At*. As you collect pictures you'll start to see a pattern of what motivates you, and what excites you. What do you do with these images? Refer to them whenever you need a reminder or pick-me-up. Or use them for your vision board, SoulCollage® card, or collage art. Or tape them around your house like on your mirror, fridge, or door.

You can take this idea further by having multiple folders for subcategories like My Perfect Home, Travel Ideas, Things That Make Me Smile, or My Perfect Mate.

Keep a second folder for handouts, cutout phrases, newsletters, and articles. Label this folder something like *Words for Me, These Words Matter to Me,* or *Open for a Pick-Me-Up.* Again, refer to these whenever you need to be re-educated or need a shot of inspiration.

When going through your folders, recycle what doesn't serve you any longer or what has lost meaning for you. We change and so does the information we need.

Dream Journal

Dreams are wild. They're curious. They're weird. They're sexual. They're scary. They're unique and special. A dream journal is exactly what you think it might be. When you wake up, pick up your journal and write what you remember. Also include details of things that really stick out for you like certain colors, people, or feelings. Patterns may appear. You can then see how your dreams correlate with what's going on in your life, and you might be able to get some insight into what you need to change and how to do it. As American playwright Marsha Norman says, "Dreams are illustrations from the book your soul is writing about you."

There are also therapists and counselors who specialize in dream analysis who can help answer the perennial question, "What the heck did that dream mean?"

A friend of mine had a recurring dream of sinking. But as she made changes in her life, her dream's ending changed. Instead of continuing to sink, she became aware that she was able to escape. What a powerful metaphor!

Asking the RIGHT questions

Debbie Ford is a popular author and motivational workshop facilitator. While I don't agree with everything she writes about, a lot of her ideas are intelligent, heartfelt, and inspirational. Her book, *The Right Questions: Ten Essential Questions to Guide You to an Extraordinary Life,* was crucial to the beginning segment of my personal, and consequently, my professional development. Below are three of the ten questions she presents that will help you know yourself better and guide you in making decisions.

> 1. Will this choice propel me toward an inspiring future or will it keep me stuck in the past?
> 2. Will this choice bring me long-term fulfillment or will it bring me short-term gratification?

3. Am I standing in my own power or am I trying to please another?

When faced with a decision, no matter how big or small, reflecting on these questions can help you. Let's suppose you're trying to lose a few pounds. One evening at dinner your friend asks, "Want to split the brownie sundae?"

Let's review Ford's three questions while considering this scenario. Question #1 – Eating this sundae will keep you stuck in the past of being overweight. Question #2 – Eating the sundae will bring you short-term gratification because it'll be yummy but it will not fulfill your desire to lose 15 pounds. Question #3 – Lastly, you don't want to offend or upset your bud, but you need to stand in your power and let her down gently by sharing your weight loss goal so she understands and can support you.

Here's another scenario. You're an aspiring actor and also work as a fitness instructor to pay the bills. Your boss at the gym hinted to you to become certified in the newest fitness program. You're not really into it but know it can bring you a bit more money eventually. You're faced with the decision: Do you use your savings for the fitness program certification because it's a perceived safer investment? Or do you take the same money to update your headshots and sign up for the stage combat class you've wanted to take for two years? Let's consider Ford's three questions again. Question #1 – The fitness certification will keep you stuck in the past because your heart is not in fitness. It is for performing. Question #2 – The certification will bring short-term gratification because you may make five dollars more an hour, but it doesn't get you closer to a full acting career. Question #3 – Lastly, your boss will be happy to offer this new program at his gym, but you'll be doing it for him and not for yourself.

Asking the RIGHT questions can change your life.

Patience of a Turtle, Vision of a Crow

There are books that get recommended to you over and over and over, year after year after year until you finally listen and go buy it. *Animal-Speak: The Spiritual & Magical Powers of Creatures Great & Small* by Ted Andrews is one of those books for me. I think I was reluctant because it seemed too woo-woo even for me. But now reading about the guides and the messages different animals have for us is quite interesting. Even if you don't believe in all this woo-woo talk, it's still pleasant and sweet to connect with animals on a deeper level and appreciate them in a whole new light.

The book is influenced by Native American animal lore and totems and will help you identify your animal totem. Do you keep seeing a yellow finch? Or images of turtles or whales? Or do elephants trigger sadness? Does a dragonfly enter your dreams often? Could you watch a squirrel for hours?   Some believe animals are messengers to us humans because they're closer to Source/Universe/God, than we are. A few of my animal guides are the red tail hawk, crow, and moose. Red tail hawk symbolizes visionary power, crow symbolizes the secret magic of creation calling, and the moose symbolizes primal feminine energies.

Maybe the animal world has some wisdom for you? To which animal(s) are you connected? Please share on the Facebook Forums! Go to www.facebook.com/NOWnoordinarywoman

CHAPTER 2

FINDING YOUR LIFE'S PURPOSE

If you engaged in all of the activities in the previous chapter of getting to know yourself a little better, you may now be thinking, "What do I do with all of this new awareness of little ol' me?" You have unique talents, skills, experiences, and passions and there's a need to live in harmony with them and to utilize them. Let me say that again but louder... YOU HAVE UNIQUE TALENTS, SKILLS, EXPERIENCES, AND PASSIONS. Many people do not believe this, or they choose to ignore this because to apply these skills and passions to their lives usually means making adjustments. Change is uncomfortable, so many choose to live in a static existence.

Finding what you're meant to be doing with your time here on Earth can be an arduous task but for some it's an easier journey. Some people know exactly what they want their roles to be and go for them. Elizabeth Gilbert, author of *Eat, Pray, Love* and her latest book *Committed* is one of these people. She avowed, "I've always considered myself lucky that I do not have many passions. There's only one pursuit that I have ever truly loved, and that pursuit is writing. This means, conveniently enough, that I never had to search for my destiny; I only had to obey it."[3]

I envy her and others like her who have one focus and don't veer from their intentions. Their lives are probably "simpler" since they don't spend a lot of time searching, trying out, frustrated, excited, disappointed, and confused about what their career should be or how they can make a living doing what they love. However, many of the women I met seem to be constant seekers – truly wanting to make a living from their passions but not yet able to find the right combination for this to manifest. The following are some ideas for you. During this time of self-discovery, having a helper or helpers, will be the key to finding your life's purpose. These helpers can be people or books and websites.

The World is Full of Helpers for You

Working with a professional on anything makes tasks more pleasurable. You go to a trained hair stylist for a haircut and to a trained yoga instructor for yoga classes. Why not go to a trained Helper to guide you with this vitally important process of finding what you're meant to do with your life? These folks have found their life's purpose, which is to help others like you clarify your ideas, gifts, fears, and desires.

---

[3] *O, The Oprah Magazine* issue November 2010

People Helpers are therapists, career counselors, life coaches, business coaches, expressive arts facilitators, expressive arts therapists, energy healers, or EFT (emotional freedom technique) practitioners.

These are some Helpers, most I personally know, who can guide you in career and life purpose clarity:

Life Coach Lisa May Simpson - Treating and preventing burnout in people who care deeply about their work.
www.lisamaysimpson.com

Intuitive Healer Christie Marie Sheldon – Are your vibrations helping or hurting you? Check out her *Love or Above*
at-home program which can help you raise your personal vibration so you can attract more good into your life! Follow the audios and workbook.
www.LoveorAbove.com

Life Coach Tamra Fleming - Dream. Decide. Do. You can live your true heart-centered life.
www.tamrafleming.com

Hand Analyst and Coach Baeth Davis - A surprisingly simple way to discover your true calling and finally uncover what has been holding you back from achieving it.
www.yourpurpose.com

Life Coach and Author Jennifer Lee – The Art of Unfolding Your Life Vision
www.artizencoaching.com

Soul Art Facilitator Laura Hollick – Mentor for New Paradigm Entrepreneurs
www.soulartstudio.com

Money, Marketing, and Soul ™ Coach Harriet Tubman Wright
www.TheWrightResort.com

Helpers who can help with your business:

Naomi Dunford and Ittybiz
www.ittybiz.com

Charlie Gilkey
www.productiveflourishings.com

Pamela Bruner
www.MakeYourSuccessEasy.com

Jo Barnes
www.thesocialnetworkingacademy.com

Lori Ruff
www.TheLinkedInDiva.com

A Truly Unique Helper

Kelly Epperson is a Happiness Coach, Author, and Speaker AND a really funny lady. Her newspaper column and weekly e-newsletter covers every day ups and downs with compassion, honesty, and great wit. She never comes across as "life is all lollipops and roses," but she embraces life's challenges with grace and humor. Her book, *365 Days of Joy*, is a pleasurable read. Her programs are titled *JOY Beyond Your Dreams* and include *JOY A.D* – after death, after divorce, and after depression. She also runs a Happiness Club near Chicago, IL.

Check her out at www.kellyepperson.com

A random side note: Speaking of joy and humor, there's an interesting organization called the AATH – Association for Applied and Therapeutic Humor. Isn't that awesome? Are you a clown, comedian, singer, humor writer and looking for a community? Or maybe you need a keynote speaker for your next event? Either way, check them out at www.aath.org.

But Be Careful of Helper-Overload and Self-Help Anxiety

Once you begin to find Helpers, Teachers, and Experts, you'll be led to more Helpers, Teachers, and Experts. At first this can be exciting because they're all so knowledgeable and inspiring. But soon, you can experience information overload. Be careful when signing up for multiple e-newsletters. All the new information and advice can overwhelm you and you can actually have an adverse reaction to it. Instead of feeling empowered by their words, you may start to feel defeated and frustrated. It may become taxing trying to complete all the action steps by these advisors. You may begin to read the success stories with exhaustion instead of enthusiasm. It can all be too much and you may experience "self-help anxiety" – when too much self-help information and advice causes anxiety instead of positivity. It may be wise to follow a few Helpers, Teachers, or Experts at a time. You can always unsubscribe to their emails and find someone new. Additionally, be careful not to compare your life to these folks. Everyone is on a different path.

Shiny Object Syndrome

Shiny object syndrome is like when a cat bounces around and follows the light from a flashlight. Oh, look it's over here, now it's over there. This syndrome seems to be prevalent among hyper-creative (HC) people. Hyper-creatives can't stop the ideas from coming in and they usually have many interests too. They go from one project to another because the next project is shiny – it's alluring because it's new! But the first project doesn't get completed. Idea creation is more stimulating than the actual grind of the work. Overwhelm sets in because they have too much on their to-do list. Sometimes HCs career hop because there are so many roles to try on or it's difficult finding the right fit for their gifts and interests. Frequently switching focus may end in feeling lost. For example, you may decide to become a virtual assistant (VA) because you love the idea of working from home. Then in your Qi Gong class the instructor announces she's offering training for certification course and you think, this is awesome. I want to share this with the world. But then a Bach Flower Remedies instructor is in town and you want to take the training course because you believe in the products. So you've decided to be a virtual assistant, Qi Gong master and give advice on using Bach Flower Remedies. Phew! That's a lot. If you really want to do it all, you can, but try to do one thing at a time. How do you choose? Refer back to Chapter 1, Know Thyself for finding answers. It takes a lot of time and energy to build a business. But once you do, then you can tackle your next idea. Consequently by the time you feel good about this first business, you may not want to pursue the others because you feel content and accomplished.

Something else to be aware of: do not get caught up in wanting to become something because it helped you. For instance, you want to become a Zumba fitness instructor because you have fun in your class and your instructor is in great shape. But is wellness and body toning a true passion that you can dedicate time, money, and energy to it for the next several years? Anything you decide to do takes time, money and energy and you don't want to just throw all of your resources all over the place and end up tired, frustrated, or unable to progress. Be aware of the next shiny object!

What are Sports Quotes Doing Here?

It may surprise you that two inspiring life purpose quotes are from the sports world!

"You miss 100% of the shots you don't take," said hockey legend Wayne Gretzky. For him there is literal meaning to this statement since he was paid to put the puck into the goal. But there's also metaphoric meaning in Gretzky's truism – if you don't try whatever your heart and gut desire, you'll never know what you are capable of achieving. If you don't ask that guy out to dinner, sing at karaoke, go to couples' counseling, take the student loan for school...you'll never know what could have been. Now I'm not saying do whatever, whenever. Proceed with caution. Most people don't try something because of fear of failure, rejection, and embarrassment. If things don't go as you wished when you attempted them, instead of looking at the negative side of it, you can think of it as a learning experience and now you have new knowledge to proceed toward your goals.

This next quote has stuck with me since high school. "Keep your eye on the ball, not on Babe Ruth." I use this quote often but I do not know who said it. It's beneficial for you to have mentors. It's natural to want to emulate someone's talents or accomplishments. But there comes the time to do your own work and make things happen for yourself. This means you need to keep fine-tuning your skills, talents, and contributions. How much time are you spending on reading books, blogs, joining programs versus working on your goals and being productive? For instance, if you're a struggling clothing designer it may be because you're spending too much time looking at award-winning designers' websites or perusing the industry's top design magazines when it might make more sense to work on your own portfolio. Getting inspiration from outside sources is one thing. But being more interested in their accomplishments than your own advancement and work is another. So keep your eye on your work, not on the work of others. Then maybe you'll become the next Babe Ruth in your field. Hey, it could happen!

Your Brain Power: Reticular Activating System

Think of a brain. There's the stem that connects the brain to the spinal cord. Inside the stem is the reticular activating system or RAS. This little guy is amazing. Because of him, we don't go crazy by hearing or attending to all the sounds and vibes around us. It's because RAS acts as a filter. Imagine if all the stimuli we hear, see, and touch throughout one day would reach our conscious, thinking mind; we would be burnt out on overload. All the house sounds, people talking, appliances buzzing, radio, planes flying by, cars and trucks, television shows, and on and on would drain our brain power. Instead, RAS acts as a gatekeeper. It shuts out the not so important and brings the important to your attention. Say you were at a crowded amusement park with lots of different sights, sounds, smells happening. You're not attuned to each one. But if someone calls your name over the noise, you'd perk up because RAS allows the familiar sound of your name to reach your conscious mind. Another example would be if you were at a party and there was background music on but you don't hear any of the songs because you're engaged in conversation. But when one of your favorite jams comes on, you definitely hear it and get your groove on.

According to Ben Greenstein and Adam Greenstein authors of *Color Atlas of Neuroscience: neuroanatomy and neurophysiology*...

The reticular activating system serves not only to maintain consciousness, but also to highlight attention to certain sensory inputs. This is achieved mainly through its inputs to the thalamus, which in turn activate certain cerebrocortical areas to focus attention on a particular sensory stimulus...The reticular activating system is also a regulator of the degree of activation allowed to reach the cerebral cortex. The diffuse direct reticulocortical inputs and those from the thalamus are in some way gated so that the cortex does not receive too intense a level of stimulation...

Another role for RAS is acting as an antenna and this is where it can help with finding your life's purpose and reaching goals. By being a gatekeeper, it keeps out information we don't need. By being an antenna, it brings to us what we do need and desire. If you set goals, make a vision board, use visualizations, have positive thoughts, or make an action plan, your brain will help you find the desired outcomes because it will now be aware of your needs. You're saying to your brain, "Hey Big Brain, if there's anything related to my goal or desire to find my life's purpose, make sure I notice it."

Say you're shopping for a new car and have a specific model in mind. You'll begin to notice more of them on the street, be aware of sales, and actually listen to the car ads on television because your

RAS is now programmed to let that info in. Same goes with finding your life purpose. Once you decide and truly set the intention that you want to find and live your purpose, then more information and opportunities will come to you like meeting the right person at a networking event, doing the right things to get the promotion, or education/training programs will seem to fall into your lap all because the repetition of your intention has programmed the RAS to let in the proper information.

The Answers Could Be As Close As Your Fingertips

Look at your fingertips. Look a little closer and you'll see swirled line patterns that are your fingerprints. Isn't it amazing that we all have fingerprints? Even more interesting is that there are different types of fingerprints and each person has a unique set of prints. We do not inherit our prints from our parents like we do our hair color and eye color. Our prints are truly unique to us.

Non-predictive hand analysis looks at your fingerprints to reveal your life's purpose and life's lesson. In addition, a trained hand analyst will also look at your hand shape, finger lengths, and special marks called gift markers, in order to give you a comprehensive reading. You can learn more about this science and find a list of trained readers through the International Institute of Hand Analysis - www.handanalysis.net.

My mini reading showed my life purpose as *artist/creative plus leader in joyous service* or *artistic leader with heart*. Part of my lesson is to work through my fear of failure and rejection.

If you'd like to read more about this topic and decipher your own hands and fingertips, these two books are available *Lifeprints: Deciphering Your Life Purpose from Your Fingerprints* by Richard Unger and *Destiny at Your Fingertips: Discover the Inner Purpose of Your Life & What It Takes to Live It* by Ronelle Coburn.

Your Tombstone Photo – Eerie or Motivating?

One of the trained hand analysts listed with the above mentioned International Institute of Hand Analysis is Baeth Davis[4]. In addition to being a gifted hand reader, she also trains others how to read hands, and is a life and business coach/motivator. Her e-newsletter provides insights about life and business and is a joy to read. She's incredibly passionate about her work but also about helping others. Some may find her honesty a bit too harsh but she always speaks from a place of compassion. On one of her free calls, she shared that she has a picture of a tombstone in her office. On the tombstone is her name, the year she was born with a dash next to it, and an open space for the year she will pass away. Is it morbid? I think it's inspiring. It might be the nudge (or kick in the ass) some people need. The reminder is that *this* is it; this one life is

---

[4] www.yourpurpose.com

what we have to live our purpose. How are you making the most of it? By whining? By living? By learning? By watching TV? By living vicariously through others like celebrities or your children? Imagine all that went into getting you here on this planet. The chances of it happening are mind-bending. You are special. Biology says so. As the tombstone picture shows, you're here for a finite amount of time. Find your purpose and start living anew. Maybe making your own headstone and epitaph will help you decide on how you want to be remembered and what you want to accomplish.

Strong Interest Inventory – What's Your Code?

Career testing offers invaluable information about you for your career, education, hobbies, happiness, and life purpose.

The Strong Interest Inventory (SII) is a test that is based on John Holland's theory, which states that there are six personality types:

1. Realistic – physical, mechanical ingenuity and dexterity
2. Investigative – researching, analyzing, writing
3. Artistic – artistic expression, musical abilities, creativity
4. Social – people skills, verbal and listening abilities
5. Enterprising – ability to motivate and direct others
6. Conventional – finances, attention to detail, data analysis

Most people are a combination of these six types. Finding out which combo of these types you are, can guide you in your quest to fulfilling work.

The SII test focuses on interests, not abilities or skills, and provides excellent feedback about possible careers and preferred work environments. This information will help you identify career and education options, understand aspects of your personality and aid in your decision-making process. The ultimate goal is to help you find work that is fulfilling, rather than merely a way to earn money.

For instance, let's say you're great with numbers so you, and others in your life, assumed you'd go into accounting or something similar. However, you have absolutely no interest in it. What kind of job satisfaction (and life satisfaction) will you have two years into the job? Or even 6 months into the job?

The SII is a multiple-choice test completed online or by a mail-in test. If you take the written test, you'll receive a report about a week later. The nine-page report provides your unique 3-letter code, which indicates the combination of the six types you are. For example, your code could be ASE (artistic, social, enterprising) or IRS (investigative, realistic, social). The report offers detailed career suggestions, including specific work environments, whether you'd flourish working in groups or independently, and more.

Many career counselors can provide this test for you. It is also available on this book's website www.NoOrdinaryWoman.net or at www.facebook.com/NOWnoordinarywoman. Then click on the shop link on the left side. I had to take the SII test for a graduate school class. It was a tremendous relief when I received my code of ASI - artistic, social, investigative. I left a secure job in order to pursue an unusual and not well-known Master's degree in expressive arts therapy and this code is one of the codes for this profession. Receiving this code validated my life-changing decision.

Also this code explains why I'm enjoying writing this book so much! I'm exercising my **A**rtistic/creative side through writing. It will be shared with others and I hope to meet new people either live or through the Facebook discussion forums, so there's the **S**ocial aspect as well. Lastly, the book is like a big research project so it's satisfying my **I**nvestigative side of seeking and researching for answers.

CHAPTER 3

BEING A MAMA

Motherhood. It's wonderful. It's tiring. It's life-enriching. It's gross. It's fulfilling. It's stressful. It's everything all at once. It is also the area of your life that takes time and effort to be conscious and present.

Supportive Resources

When I was pregnant I naturally sought out a supportive community. I was living in a new town (again) and family and friends were far away. Also, my sister's and my friends' children were already in kindergarten and grade school. I needed to be around women who were also pregnant and beginning their motherhood journey.

I found such a community online at www.Mothering.com, which is a website for natural family living. Even though its core is "natural family living," you can find help with a variety of your mothering questions. Read what other moms have done or ask questions in the forums. The discussion topics are plentiful such as planning birthday parties, meal planning, special needs, using a midwife or a birthing tub, natural remedies for parents, kids and pets, breastfeeding help, keeping sons intact (i.e., to circumcise or not to circumcise), proper essential oil use, and much more.

I personally used the forums to learn more about cloth diapering, preparing my body for birthing, vaccination education, and learned about WAHMs (Work at Home Moms), and how other moms try to balance family and career.

I also ended up finding a wonderful group through this site called Holistic Moms Network (HMN), which is a national nonprofit with groups that meet locally on a monthly basis. When I moved, yet again, I connected with my local HMN group and ended up being a volunteer leader for a year and a half.

Surround yourself with support, there's nothing like getting answers from mamas who have been there.

Make Music Together

Early exposure to music can help your child's development. Research shows that music can increase a child's self-confidence, verbal and memory skills, and spatial-temporal reasoning. Introducing them to a wide variety of music exposes them to different beats and making up songs helps with their imagination and musical development. All of this is positive enrichment for your child. Music at home can include filling a container with beans or rice for shakers, banging on pots and pans for drums, or humming.

If you want to take a class, there are a variety of music classes available for young children. Music Together is one example. A Music Together class is exciting and wholesome. Class begins with parents or caregivers and children sitting on the floor in a circle singing the welcome song. Some classes involve dancing with colorful scarves and playing an assortment of handheld percussive instruments. At times large drums are used, like gathering drums, which sit on the floor and are big enough for four children. With all of this sound and energy, the classes are contained and very sweet. It's interesting to see weekly changes in the kids. It's also nice to meet other families who share your interest in music exposure for young children. In my experience, the trained teachers are patient and understand that music exposure is more important than obedient participation or singing precise lyrics.

I loved the Music Together classes as much as my son did. The songs are still in our repertoire and he occasionally sings them when playing alone. We started with a baby's class at six months old. The babies observed and listened and it appeared the rhythms and lyrics were being processed.

Some Music Together classes are intergenerational and held in nursing homes or assisted living facilities. So the elders get to be part of the music-making class as well. How enriching for them!

Nonviolent Communication

Do you ever think there's got to be a more loving and effective way to communicate with your children and to model a positive communication style?

Nonviolent communication (NVC) may be a solution. It's based on four stages: observation, feeling, need, and request. When I observe _____, I feel _____ because I have a need for _____. Would you (be willing to) _____?

Here are a couple scenarios to explain how I think it works.

Scenario #1
Your child hits your other child. You can approach the situation by stating, "When I <u>observe</u> you hitting your younger brother, I <u>feel</u> sad because I have a <u>need</u> for a loving family and a calm household. <u>Would you</u> be willing to be a respectful and understanding big brother and ask nicely for your toy next time?"

Now here's the same scenario without sounding like it's from a textbook: "Hey Nestor, I just <u>saw</u> you hit Constantine. Hitting makes me <u>feel</u> sad and Constantine sad, too. We all <u>want</u> to feel safe and comfortable in our home and hitting isn't allowed. Next time <u>could you</u> ask him for the toy? He's a lot younger than you, and he doesn't understand sharing yet."

Scenario #2

Your 16 year old is late for curfew. Using NVC, you can react to the situation by stating, "When I <u>observe</u> you coming in 35 minutes late after curfew, I <u>feel</u> like you don't respect me, and I have a <u>need</u> for us to trust each other and have a loving family environment. <u>Would you</u> be willing to come home on time?"

Let's translate that to real life: "<u>Look at the clock</u> Sabina, it's 35 minutes passed curfew. I <u>feel</u> like you're not respecting the curfew that we agreed was fair, and I <u>need</u> you to understand that I worry when you're late, and I <u>need</u> to feel like I can trust you. Next time, <u>will you</u> come home on time so I can trust you again?"

Let's review the stages and scenarios.

Stage 1 Observation – the concrete action, not the interpretation but what actually happened.

Scenario #1 - Nestor hit his younger brother.

Scenario #2 - Sabina was late.

Stage 2 Feeling – observe your own feelings and take responsibility for them. I feel...because. Not "You make me feel..."

Scenario #1 - I feel sad *because* I don't like violence.

Scenario #2 - I feel disrespected *because* our agreement was not honored and my trust is shaky if not broken.

Stage 3 Need – State your need from the situation.

Scenario #1 - I need to have a safe, violent-free household.

Scenario #2 - I need to trust my teenager.

Stage 4 Request – Make a request so the other person understands the situation and what will placate the situation.

Scenario #1 - Can you be patient with your younger brother and ask for the toy next time using your words instead of what happened earlier?

Scenario #2 - Can you come home at the agreed upon curfew time so we can maintain the trust?

The Center for Non-violent Communication is a good resource for more ideas and also a good place to find local workshops and classes.

Multiple Intelligences

In my early twenties, over a decade before I was a parent, I worked with children as an environmental educator in an overnight weeklong camp setting. I witnessed how the "problem" kids, usually boys, did really well on the hikes and enjoyed learning the night sky, different birds, and the names of deciduous trees. These "problem" kids never gave me any trouble. Actually, I never really had any issues with any of the kids. I suspect it was because they were out of school, in nature, free to move around, and having fun. But the so-called problem kids and the kids who were diagnosed with ADHD stood out to me. Upon arrival, the teachers would take me aside and tell me which kids to watch out for. I never saw the anticipated bad behavior and instead witnessed these kids engaged and asking really great questions. I realized then that kids all learn differently and I questioned traditional schooling and testing, where everyone must conform to certain standards. What if a child can name 50 trees by inspecting their leaves and needles but doesn't do so well in a biology class? Does that make him dumb or a bad student? Are we setting up the children who learn differently for constant failure because their learning styles aren't in sync with the school system? Many years later, I got some answers about learning styles.

Dr. Howard Gardner, a developmental psychologist, created the theory of multiple intelligences. The theory of multiple intelligences explains that humans learn and process information differently. We, as parents, can use this information to understand ourselves and our children better. Depending on your child, the information may be useful to overcome learning obstacles. Or it will help you be aware of what makes your child tick. According to the theory, we all possess the eight intelligences listed below but in different amounts. Some outweigh the others, which isn't good or bad. It just is.

The eight different intelligences[5] are:

Verbal/Linguistic – word smart

These children (and adults) tend to do well with words, written or spoken. They enjoy reading, writing, telling stories, debating, and giving speeches. Careers paths may include author, researcher, reporter, poet, teacher, saleperson, comedian, librarian, or motivational speaker.

Logical/Mathematical – number smart

These kids tend to be good with numbers and planning. They enjoy mathematics and puzzles. Career paths may include auditor, lawyer, physician, detective, or computer programmer.

Interpersonal – people smart

These kids tend to be extroverts and tend to be aware of other people's moods and feelings. They cooperate easily, communicate effectively and are empathetic. They enjoy groups, board games, and community involvement. They are often good leaders and flourish in the helping fields. Career paths may include actor, social worker, restaurateur, or marketing specialist.

---

[5] www.best-career-match.com/career-chart.html

Intrapersonal – myself smart

These kids tend to be introverts and prefer to work alone. They understand their emotions and goals. They tend to perform at high levels and often show signs of perfectionism. Journaling, independent study, and individual games are often of interest. Career paths may include philosopher, energy healer, therapist, artist, or criminologist.

Musical – music smart

These kids are interested in tones, rhythms, and singing. They typically are sensitive or attuned to sounds and music. They remember things in rhythm or rhyme. Career paths may include speech pathologist, disc jockey, sound editor, musician, or music therapist.

Visual/spatial – picture smart

Kids here have strong visual memories, are often artistically inclined, may have a good sense of direction, and have good eye-hand coordination. Career paths may include architect, artist, interior designer, pilot, webmaster, film animator, or mechanic.

Naturalistic – nature smart

These kids like animals, nature, and they tend to nurture and grow things. They are good at recognizing species or enjoy gardens, aquariums, binoculars, telescopes, terrariums, and ant farms.

Career paths may include veterinarian or vet assistant, meteorologist, gardener, dog trainer, environmental lawyer, marine biologist, or ecologist.

Body/Kinesthetic – body smart

These kids lean towards moving, being action-oriented, sports, dancing, gymnastics, construction and deconstruction, digging, performing, creative movement, and cooking. Career paths may include athlete, firefighter, recreational therapist, surgeon, or yoga instructor.

Which intelligences describe for your kids? How can you use this new information of their intelligences to be a more conscious parent?

Role Model

This isn't groundbreaking news: You are your child's primary role model. If you yell, they'll learn to yell. If you give hugs, they'll probably give hugs. If you hit, they're more likely to hit others. Children are little sponges that absorb everything from their environment. One day, I repeatedly told my son, who was three at the time that he couldn't have something that was on the table. But he continued to reach and ask for it until he finally almost grabbed it. Without thinking, I grabbed his hand, squeezed, and sternly said, "No! You cannot have that!" The loudness of my voice and the squeeze scared him and the tears came. After the tears subsided we discussed the incident, so that we both understood what happened and what could have happened differently. The next day, our dog was in his way, and he got frustrated. Guess what he did to remedy the situation? Yep, he grabbed her tail, squeezed, and sternly said, "NO!!!!" The dog yelped, I yelled, and again more tears. So we had to talk about this incident.

I felt badly about my poor role modeling. If I'd never shown him how to get frustrated and squeeze, he wouldn't have done it. He never did it before and he hasn't done it since. But I remember this every every time I need to be reminded that I'm one of his main role models...both for good behavior and not-so-good behavior. So Mamas check yourself when your kid is whining, bossy, and short-tempered...does it emit from you?

Celebrate Half Birthdays

Remember when you were young and you'd proudly announce you were nine...*and a half*! That half meant you were getting older and wiser. With kids it's fun to celebrate halves because you're keenly aware how fast they're growing, changing, and aging. It allows you to be mindful, to be thankful, and to be present for your child. It doesn't mean you have to rent a bounce house or buy balloons to celebrate. Celebrate by marking their height against the wall, or make half birthday cupcakes, which are actually cut in half, or just acknowledging it with a big hug.

Celebrating half birthdays can be fun for adults, too. Again, it's about being mindful of the time passing. This can be a time to pat yourself on the back for completing a goal (finally fixed the roof) or for enduring a life challenge (divorce). It might be a good time to add a few pages in your gratitude journal or create a new vision board.

Teen Brains

It seems like many adults forget children aren't mini adults and expect them to act as if they know what to do. It's the same with teenagers—they still aren't adults. A teenager's body might be saying "I'm almost an adult," but their emotions and reasoning say something else because their brains aren't fully developed yet. So remember this tidbit when they mess up, have mood swings, and don't use their best judgment.

Inside the teen brain: Behavior can be baffling when young minds are taking shape[6], is an article by S. Brownlee, R. Hotinski, B.

---

[6] US News and World Report in AUGUST 9, 1999

Pailthorp, E. Ragan, and K. Wong, explaining this further:

> *Yes, teenagers do have brains, but theirs don't yet function like an adult's. With the advent of technologies such as magnetic resonance imaging, neuroscientists have discovered that the adolescent brain is far from mature. "The teenage brain is a work in progress," says Sandra Witelson, a neuroscientist at McMaster University in Ontario, and it's a work that develops in fits and starts. Until the past decade, neuroscientists believed that the brain was fully developed by the time a child reached puberty and that the 100 billion neurons, or nerves, inside an adult's skull--the hardware of the brain—were already in place by the time pimples began to sprout. The supposition was that a teenager could think like an adult if only he or she would cram in the necessary software--a little algebra here, some Civil War history there, capped by proficiency in balancing a checkbook. But the neural circuitry, or hardware, it turns out, isn't completely installed in most people until their early 20s.*

And just as a teenager is all legs one day and all nose and ears the next, different regions of his brain are developing on different timetables. For instance, one of the last parts to mature is in charge of making sound judgments and calming unruly emotions.

This article confirms that your teenager teeters frequently between being a naïve sensitive child and being a self-sufficient adult. It's a confusing time for everyone. But with this new information, you can be more aware about what's sinking in and what isn't when it comes to them understanding directions, consequences, and outcomes.

CHAPTER 4

YOUR MOOLAH

Cash. Cheddar. Dough. You need it. You want it. Part of conscious living is your financial flow. It cannot be ignored, no matter how much you have.

Treat Your Financials Like a Friend

When bills show up in your mailbox, do you huff, curse a little, then toss them in a pile and ignore them? If one of your friends showed up on your doorstep, would you huff, curse, and ignore them? I hope not. I'm assuming you'd welcome them in and find out what's going on and treat them with respect. This treatment could be applied to your money and bills.

By not opening your monthly financial statements or bills, you're not living consciously and instead you're living in fear, not being responsible, and not respecting your money. You're ignoring a very big part of your life, something you need and most likely want more of it. How will more money come to you if you can't manage what you have now? You may need to find a solution to your debt and, in addition, you may need to find a solution to your anxiety around money. Both of these are discussed later.

One way to treat your debt or bills as a friend is to give it proper attention by opening the mail, organizing the bills, and get a system established. Another way to give it attention is to write "Thank You" on the invoices or the checks paying the bills. If you pay a bill on the internet, you can write "Thank You" on that particular day in your calendar. This activity helps you remember why you are giving your money away at that particular moment and embracing the gratitude that comes forth. "Thank you" for the car I drive. "Thank you" for the electricity that allows me to cook indoors. "Thank you" for the medical treatment I received. "Thank you" for the clothing I just bought. Whom are you thanking? You are acknowledging the people and systems that gave you credit or a loan, the utility facilities and the people who provide the services, and the banks for trusting you with a mortgage. This teeny act helps you to be aware of how much you have and how your money is being used to provide the life you choose to live. Again, you're thinking of your financials as a friend. You'd thank your friend for giving you something. Well, you're financial responsibilities are giving you something as well.

Once you have a mindful relationship with your money, bills, debt, and investments, do you think there's a chance it will blossom?

Try This Easy Empowering Step & Train Your Brain

List all of your monthly expenses. After you pay them, cross them off – preferably in red or a bright color. We all love to accomplish things. Doesn't it feel good to cross off items on your to-do list? This is the same idea. Crossing off the payments for heat, trash removal, mortgage, rent, and tuition instills a sense of pride. You've proved you're responsible and serious about money management. You can see your accomplishments and feel good about them.

This repeated activity trains your brain to think that you are capable of earning money, being responsible with it, and that you get things done. Therefore, you are capable of going to the next level with your earnings and bills. You're empowered to expand!

What's Your Magic Number?

If you're like most people, you'd prefer to have more money because life would be better, easier, and more pleasurable. How much more do you need to reach a level of pure contentment? What is your monthly magic number? How much do you want to earn/receive/need per month to make you happy? For this exercise, you don't have to know from where the money will come.

You're just becoming aware of exactly how much money would allow you to be really content and comfortable. Take into account such things as living expenses, gifts, retirement, vacations, savings, debt, education, and big purchases like cars and vacation homes. Once you know this exact number, then you can begin to make advances towards it. Talking with your partner, a life coach, a financial planner, or a business coach may help you get to that magic number. But right now, not being clear about your money target is probably making your goals more difficult to attain than they need to be.

Attack the Lack Mindset

A lack mindset is living with limiting beliefs about money, opportunities, and resources. It can include thoughts that you're not worthy of more; or you *must* work hard to make ends meet. Another aspect of a lack mindset is thinking, *why should I have more when there are so many others with less?* Having a lack mindset may be keeping you from reaching your potential because you continually focus on scarcity, fears, and negativity.

How do you think about money? What are your money beliefs? What's been ingrained in you from childhood? What did you hear your parents or caregivers say about money? *Work hard. Money doesn't grow on trees. Poor people will try to take from you.*

Wealthy people are snobs. The almighty dollar is king. Any of these sound familiar?

Your money beliefs come from childhood. If there was a focus on scarcity when you were young chances are it's manifested as an adult. About five years ago, my lack mindset affected my paintings. I bought these lovely, expensive, high quality paints. Due to my limiting mindset, I was afraid to explore with them in my work because I coveted them. I didn't want to "waste" them. I was afraid I wasn't going to be able to afford more so I didn't really use them. Look at the words I just used...*coveted, waste, afraid.* These are full of negativity. Not surprising, my art suffered. Every time I looked at the paints on my table, my lack mindset was triggered. Even before I picked up my paintbrush, I was not in a good space to create. Since my art suffered, my spirit suffered because I wasn't producing art I enjoyed. Well, if anyone creates anything, from paintings to scrapbooking to gardening to glasswork to creative writing, there's always "waste" in the process. You usually don't use everything you have. Part of the creative process is trimming, deleting, cutting, and tossing. In order to explore, test, and take risks, you must use your supplies. Even if you're not sure if it's going to work out and be part of a finished product, it has to be okay with you to chalk it up to a learning experience. It took me months (maybe years) to grasp and accept this concept and believe that I will be able to replace the high quality paints when needed.

A surprising example of some folks with lack mindsets are those with inheritances and trust funds. I know recipients of gifted money and they are frequently afraid to expand and develop their personal potential because the security blanket of their financial accounts actually holds them back. Since the money was given to them, they feel they have to be responsible with it, and hold on to it as tight as possible. Why? It may be because they're afraid they could never make this large sum of money on their own and/or they feel this is it and there's no more. Again, this is an example of a fear-based belief. Thus they take no risks because they fear losing their funds. Someone in their life, usually someone that loves them very much, probably worked hard to provide this money cushion for them; consequently, they can't use it for anything beyond basic living or education. They can't be "irresponsible" with this gift because that would be disrespectful to the person who gave it them. So it's surprising to hear that even financially comfortable people who pay their bills on time, have healthy saving accounts, investments and education, can still have a lack mindset.

In order to move past your lack mindset, you'll need help. This help can come by way of books or people. Some women who have lived with a lack mindset and struggled but changed their lives and the lives of thousands of women (and some men) are Kendall

Sumerhawk, Christine Kane, and Ali Brown.[7] You'll be inspired by their stories and learn more about getting over your lack mindset.

Got Debt?

Debt is like a rain cloud following you around but it can be managed. Here are two ways to approach your debt, so you can see the light at the end of the tunnel.

The first idea is the debt snowball plan. Below are the steps from www.GetRichSlowly.org, which is paraphrasing Dave Ramsey's book, *The Total Money Makeover:*

1. Order your debts from lowest to highest balance.
2. Designate a certain amount of money to pay toward debts each month.
3. Pay the minimum payment on all debts except the one with the lowest balance.
4. Throw every penny you can at the debt with the lowest balance.
5. When that debt is gone, do not alter the monthly amount used to pay your debts, but throw all you can at the debt with the next lowest balance.

First, you've decided to no longer use your credit cards and will not add any more debt to them. You've designated $80 per month

---

[7] www.kendallsummerhawk.com, www.christinekane.com, www.alibrown.com

to go towards your two credit card debts. Your minimum monthly payment for Credit Card #2, the larger debt of the two cards, is $30. As you can see from the rudimentary chart, in August you're going to kick up your payment for Credit Card #2 because Credit Card #1 is all gone. Yay! Now, with your first debt out of the way, use that $50 towards the next debt to pay it down faster. You do not adjust your monthly $80 payment even though one credit card is paid off.

	June	July	Aug	Sept	Oct
Credit Card #1 With $100 balance	$50	$50	---	---	---
Credit Card #2 with $1,200 balance	$30	$30	$80	$80	$80
Money to pay off Credit Cards per month	$80	$80	$80	$80	$80

A second approach to your debt repayment is to work with a debt consolidation center. I used one of them in my early 30s to manage debt that I created in my 20s from paying for college textbooks, tuition, and traveling. A manageable personal program was created with a financial counselor and I became free of consumer debt (credit cards, not federal student loans) in a couple of years. The process helped me not feel overwhelmed. Instead it increased my confidence and helped improve my credit score. Fast forward ten years later, I applied for a small business loan and was accepted because I had completed a debt consolidation plan. I assumed this looked favorably to the loan officers because it proved I took my financial responsibilities seriously.

One way to find an agency near you is to go to the National Foundation for Credit Counseling at www.nfcc.org.

Money Is Energy

The movie *Twenty Bucks* came out in the early 90s. Have you seen it? The storyline follows a single 20-dollar bill as it travels from hand to hand. It goes from the ATM to a bakery to a stripper at a bachelor party to an herbal remedy lady and so on and so on. There's energy on that bill. Money is a kind of energy and we humans are conduits for energy. Energy passes through us and moves on to other people, animals, and things.

In Maria Nemeth's book, *The Energy of Money*, she explains how we are conduits for money energy. Infinite energy comes into us and through us, or at least it tries to, and often results in our goals and dreams. But "money sludge" and "money leaks" gunk up the money flow. Money sludge is unpaid debts, credit card balances, not making a will, and the like. Money leaks are ways we unconsciously spend money. This is so easy to do nowadays with debit cards, credit cards, and Paypal accounts. Nemeth suggests finding our money leaks, which are essentially energy leaks because money is energy, and patch them up. She suggests tracking every cent you spend for the next thirty days. This will reveal where the leaks are. You can do it yourself, or if you have a family you can get them involved as well. This isn't about changing your spending habits at this time. It's about becoming aware and conscious of where your money/energy is going. Then you can begin to make appropriate decisions and plans after evaluating the results.

Years before reading Nemeth's book, I did a version of this exercise in my early 30s to see where my money was going just on alcoholic drinks. During this time of my life, I didn't have a child and lived in a Chicago neighborhood with fantastic bars, restaurants, and music venues. For about three weeks, I withheld from drinking and tracked every time I *would have* had a drink and the money I saved. The numbers added up quickly. $140 was the estimated amount saved by the end of the experiment. If I kept it up I could have possibly saved $1,000-$2,000 that year. I was astonished because I complained all the time that I didn't have a lot of money in my savings account or I didn't have "extra" money for any self-care treats like a massage or pedicure. The fact was my savings and massages were going towards happy hours (that weren't really happy, more like bitch fests after work), fancy expensive brunch drinks, and beer at home to drink after work or with visiting friends.

Nowadays my alcohol consumption is minimal to non-existent so I guess I'm saving money now. But I wasted so much back then.

You're in the Marketing Funnel

Since you purchase goods and services, you are a consumer. As a consumer, you are part of marketing funnels and you should be aware of it. We'll discuss one example of an online marketing funnel. A funnel is wide at the top and narrow at the bottom. At the top of this online marketing funnel are freebies. When you go to a website, there's usually something free for you as long as you provide your email address. Freebies are ebooks, cds, pdfs, book chapter, song, meditation, newsletters, and how to videos. Now that the website owner has your email address, you will then be introduced to their products and/or services through future emails. The hope is that you test the waters and begin to trust them with the freebie and e-newsletter. Then purchase a low cost item. If impressed with the freebie and low cost item eventually you may pay for higher cost products or services. The funnel depicts the progression of how a lot of people/leads come in for the freebie but the number of buyers will get less and less as the products become more and more expensive.   You, the consumer, slides down the funnel if you find value in this product or service.

First you sign up for a free book chapter. Then you may

purchase the book. After that, you may go to the author's workshop. Many people will download the freebie. Less will buy the book and only those who feel a real connection will invest in the workshop.

On the flip side, if you are a business owner, utilizing this marketing strategy may be lucrative for you. What can you offer as a freebie to convert website visitors to buying prospects?

Now, there is nothing wrong with this marketing approach. It's not trickery. But it's useful to be aware of what you're signing up for. Definitely sign up for freebies or newsletters! It's so easy to unsubscribe if you ever want out.

Advice from a Female Financial Planner Who's Been There

Helen Georgaklis, financial planner, author, and CEO of 99 Series Publishers has experienced financial burdens and crises throughout her life. But she has come out on top despite them. Here are some words of wisdom for women of any age from her book *99 Things Women Wish They Knew Before Planning for Retirement:*

> Quote #1: *Clothing and shoes... what else is there? We can never have enough! Shopping is probably one of the best activities, especially*

when we're feeling down. The problem is that it's addictive. We will go out of our way to afford what we want—even if we're broke! How many times have you gone shopping and paid cash instead of whipping out the plastic?

The more credit you use during your working years, the less cash you will have available during your retirement. I am never one to back down from great sales in the fashion industry, especially in today's times, but at what cost? Will your shopping affect your retirement?

Read that statement again, "The more credit you are using during your working years, the less cash you will have available during retirement." Now, that's a thinker. Anytime interest is paid on your credit cards and loans, it's robbing you of future money. So the takeaway here is to either pay cash, use your debit card, or pay off your credit cards in full every month and not accrue interest.

Quote #2: *Investing for women is special because we live longer and have less accumulated pensionable earnings. This is due to the likelihood that we will take time out of the workforce, often more than once in our lives. Also, as you well know, we generally earn less than men. Every one of you should have a written financial plan explaining your investments, your different portfolios, and goals associated with each one.*

This statement really got to me. Maybe it's because I'm 40 now and have left the full-time workforce to raise my child. Since I chose to do that I have less accumulated pensionable earnings. Suppose if something happened to my marriage (I really hope that it doesn't!), I have less saved for my retirement because I've been out of the workforce. I know that is obvious but this thought never crossed my mind when I was making the decision to be a mostly stay-at-home/work-from-home kind of mom.

I had a glimpse of this reality check over a year ago when I had to purchase a new computer since my old one bit the dust. The best deal was to open an account with the store and buy through their credit card because no interest would accrue. However, I was denied an account because I haven't *worked* for over a year. The customer service rep wasn't impressed by my soliloquy of how I have *worked* for the last couple of years raising a child and working from home. He simply said I haven't had a real full-time job. Argh!

But in order for me to continue my work from home and to write this book you're holding in your hands, I *had* to have a computer. It would have been impossible to run over to the library to do my work. So...I had to turn to my hubby who had a "real" job and opened the account in his name. Oh, the frustration I felt.

So Ladies, be keenly aware when making financial decisions because it may change the layout of your future.

Why You Must Indulge

According to T. Harv Eker, author of *Secrets of the Millionaire Mind,* it's necessary to have fun and take care of yourself on a monthly basis. Here's his reason:

> *Pamper yourself. At least once a month do*
> *something special to nurture yourself and your*
> *spirit. Get a massage, a manicure, or a pedicure*
> *and take yourself for an extravagant lunch or*
> *dinner, rent a boat or a weekend cottage, have*
> *someone bring you breakfast in bed. (You*
> *might have to trade with a friend or family*
> *member). Do things that will allow you to feel*
> *rich and deserving. Again, the vibrational*
> *energy you emit from this kind of experience*

will send a message to the universe that you
live abundantly, and again, the universe will
simply do its job and say, 'okay' and give you
opportunities for more.

Do you believe this? Do you think if you live with an abundant mindset, the universe will provide more? Or is this kind of thinking self-indulgent and leads to overspending? Thinking *I am worth it* brings you joy, thus, raises your energy. You are aware that you're special and worthy of goodness. But take heed because this positive action could turn out to be a slippery slope which ends at a negative place called debt.

My little indulgence may seem silly to some but I like to purchase handcrafted, artisan cold-pressed soaps. While it's not a weekend cottage, it's an indulgence because the price is a few bucks more than regular soap and I'm passing on the flow of money energy to a small business owner. They make my skin feel wonderful and the fresh scents from the essential oils are heavenly. It's my reminder that I'm worth "luxury" even if the luxury item is bath soap.

Everyone Loves A Deal

Everyone digs a good deal and finding them is part of conscious living.

Have you heard of Blissmo? Daily deals are emailed for organic, sustainable, and environmentally-friendly items. There are deals on makeup, skincare, food, stationery, water bottles, and clothing. The site also offers the Blissmobox. For $19 per month, a box of organic and eco-friendly products is mailed to you. It's like a monthly pick-me-up!

www.blissmo.com

Just in case you don't know about Groupon I wanted to include it as well. Their daily deals include discounts at restaurants, spas, salons, printing photo books, framing, home-delivered organic groceries, photo books, even an improv class! Often restaurant deals offer something like you pay $20 for a $40 meal. So when your bill comes to the table for $49, all you need to pay is $9 with your printed Groupon. Of course, don't forget that you need to leave a tip on the $49 total, not the $9 adjusted total.

If you're a business owner, you'll be interested in this site as well. On a Thursday in March 2011, a well-known Rochester, NY salon, Scott Miller, announced a $25 pedicure. The normal price was $54, so it was a 54% discount. Guess how many people bought it? 100 people? Keep guessing! By 5:55 am the deal was on with 25 Groupons sold. Then within hours, 3,229 people bought it. By 3:12 pm, the deal sold out to a whopping 4,000 people. Yes, 4,000 people bought the deal! Groupon is free to join. Another deal-making website is www.LivingSocial.com.

Are you a golfer or know one? The Early Birdie is a deal site just for golfers in New York, New Jersey, and Connecticut. Deals include courses, teaches and other related items.

Creative Living

The future belongs to a very different kind of person with a very different kind of mind— creators and empathizers, pattern recognizers, and meaning makers. These people—artists, inventors, designers, storytellers, caregivers, consolers, big picture thinkers—will now reap society's richest rewards and share its greatest joys.

Daniel Pink, *A Whole New Mind: Why Right-Brainers Will Rule the Future*

By nature, humans are creative. We think creatively. We express ourselves. We are problem solvers, and we care about aesthetics.

In Chapter 5 Make It With Your Hands, you'll get a chance to exercise your Creative Self with eight art-making ideas. Chapter 6 Other Creative Outlets, provides cool ideas to express yourself using the other modalities of writing, music, and more. Have fun in

Chapter 7 Let The Good Times Roll with unique ideas for creative living.

CHAPTER 5

MAKE IT WITH YOUR HANDS

Small Scale Art

Staring at a large six-foot-tall painting, especially abstracts, brings me joy. It's a treat to get lost in the flow, colors, and textures. These big works of art are bold and demand attention. I remember seeing my first Jackson Pollock at the Walter's Art Gallery in Baltimore as a young adult. It was larger than any person in the room. Its energy enveloped me. I was fixated. From then on, my love for the genre grew. I also enjoy painting on such a large scale but often can't due to space. Many people don't have the creating space for such large pieces. The alternative is to go small and small can still have an impact.

Artist Trading Cards (ATCs) are the size of baseball cards (2.5 inches x 3.5 inches / 6.4 cm x 8.9 cm) and are meant to be traded just like baseball cards. I've been making ATCs for about six years. With ATCs you can make art and exercise your Creative Self without costly art supplies. Nor do you need a large studio space. Trading ATCs is also a great way to obtain original art without spending a lot of money. Since there are active communities of ATC artists and traders globally, I've traded with people from around the world. As an active member of the ATC community, you get to know people through their art processes and developments. Most art forms are accepted: paintings, drawings, abstract, realistic, figurative, mixed media, collage, computer generated, found art, even fabric art. There's a sense of validation when someone requests my ATCs, and it's a joy to request ATCs from others.

ACEOs are Art Cards, Editions and Originals and are the same size as ATCs but are meant for sale and purchase not trading.

For more information, check out ATC groups on www.Flickr.com. Here are a few awesome ATC artists on Flickr: mikesmom8, grrrdjules, Pjevsen (Denmark), tengds (Thailand), Shay NOLA, autumnsensation, JanDart, Norma Frances, Lindsaywhimsy, candy-n29, and Red Heart Studio. Other ATC websites include www.illustratedatcs.com, www.atcsforall.com, and www.artcardswanted.com.

As a side note: There are other Flickr artists worth checking out even though they do not create ATCs. These folks create digital art, paintings, photographs, and craft: April Rain Photography, M.A. Wakeley, Chopak, Yael Fran (Argentina), and Hiroshi Matsumoto (Japan).

Another small-scale art option is Art-o-mat. Art-o-mat is one of the most unique art exchanges. Clark Whittington, Founder of Art-o-Mat, takes old cigarette vending machines (remember the ones with the pull knobs?) and redesigns them to vend little blocks or boxes of art. These revamped machines are in art galleries, Whole Foods Markets, restaurants, and Las Vegas' casino hotel, The Cosmopolitan. See Whittington's cigarette machines on their Flickr page at http://www.flickr.com/photos/clarkwhittington and read more about their journeys on their blog at http://news.artomat.org.

The Art of SoulCollage®

To make a collage, one needs to assemble images, materials, or objects onto a surface. It's a fun process and at times it can be therapeutic. SoulCollage® takes the collage art form to a different level because it's an intuitive process for self-discovery. A SoulCollage card is created by gluing magazine images to heavy cardstock paper. The SoulCollage deck contains one Source card, which symbolizing the "Oneness of All Things," and at least four separate suits: The Committee Suit (The Psychological Dimension), The Community Suit (The Communal Dimension), The Companion Suit (The Energetic Dimension), and the Council Suit (The Spiritual Dimension). After you create a number of SoulCollage® cards, you'll have a deck. Pick a random card from your deck each morning to use as your guide for the day. Cards can be created at home or in a group setting.

To find a SoulCollage® facilitator near you, go to the www.soulcollage.com. To join an active online community or to purchase supplies, check out Anne Marie Bennett's website www.kaleidosoul.com. In 2010 a new edition of Seena Frost's book was published, *SoulCollage Evolving: An Intuitive Collage Process for Self-Discovery and Community*.

Hand Sculptures

Hands do many things - things you're proud of and things you're ashamed of and things you often don't reflect on. They're used to reach out for a handshake or close up for a punch. They're responsible for counting, hitchhiking, making vulgar gestures, stealing, bathing a baby, digging, tickling, helping someone up and giving high fives.

What have you done with your hands? What do you want to do with them? Honor them by creating your hand sculpture. You'll need plaster wrap strips, which can be bought at an arts and crafts store, petroleum gel, scissors, and water. It's best to have someone do this with you. Here's what you need to do:

First, cut the plaster wrap strips into a variety of sizes and get a bowl of warm water. Be sure to use a bowl that you can throw away afterwards. A plastic takeout container may work.

Next, apply the petroleum jelly to your hand and fingers so there's a barrier between you and the plaster wrap. This jelly will allow you to slip off the sculpture after it dries on your hand and fingers.

After the jelly is on, dip the plaster strips into the warm water and begin to wrap the wet strips around your fingers and hands. Be sure to keep your hand still doing this process. It will pretty much feel like a cast is going on.

After the whole hand is covered, wait a few minutes until the sculpture has hardened a little bit. But don't wait for it to be entirely rigid because it will be very difficult to remove from your hand if it's solid.

Then, cut the sculpture along the side of your hand by carefully slipping one side of the scissors into an open area near your wrist, and cut enough so you can wiggle your hand out. Cut only as much as necessary to get your hand out.

Next, apply a couple of wet plaster strips to repair where you just cut.

Finally, allow the piece to dry overnight. Once it's fully dried, you can then paint or decorate it.

I created a how-to video on this process a few years ago that will be useful to watch. See the process first before trying it yourself. Create with caution and at your own risk. To find my video, go to YouTube and search for "plaster wrap hand." Over a 1,600 views already! – wow, there're a lot of folks making hand sculptures! Yahoo!

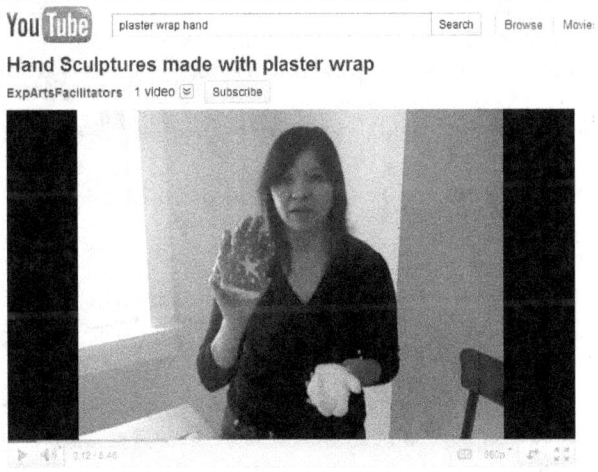

Play In The Tray – Sandtray Explorations

Imagine a wood tray about 20 inches by 30 inches (50.8 cm x 67.2 cm), with walls about four inches (10.2 cm) high. Inside the tray is black sand waiting for you to explore its coolness and soothing texture. After a guided centering exercise, you take a basket and begin collecting objects and figurines from shelves and tables. There are about 500 miniature objects to choose from – natural objects like stones and seashells, animals, people, cars, boats, household items and furniture, beads, marbles, mirrors, and much more. But only a number of these objects will interest you enough to collect it for your tray. After you finish choosing your objects, you arrange them in the tray any way you wish. After your scene is complete, you share what you just created either in your journal or with a witness like me or a friend. Sandtray Exploration is my second most popular workshop. It's usually a calm, meditative time and participants enjoy seeing and describing their scenes in the tray. This intuitive process brings in sculpture and drama elements.

In my experience, most people enjoy the sandtray process. They love this unique method of self-exploration, not to mention that almost everyone enjoys getting their hands in the sand. Children, teens, adults, and seniors can benefit from doing Sandtray Explorations.

If you wish to do this at home, you can use a medium to large plastic storage box with a lid. Collect objects of meaning or interest and create a scene. The sand can be any color - white, blue, green, red – but I use black because it's aesthetically pleasing and it helps accentuate the objects that are scattered on top of it. It's important to process the scene afterwards because each object has a different meaning to you personally. Try to relate how this scene is relevant in your life right now and incorporate the message it is relaying.

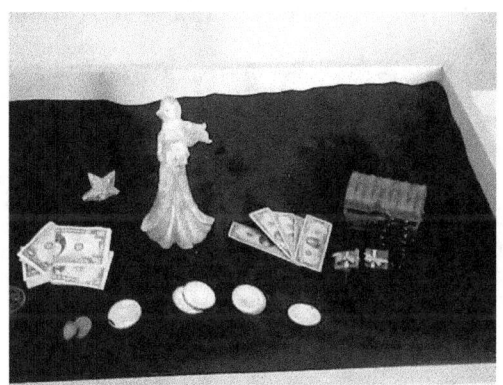

Upcycled Inspirational Art

Create unique art with an inspirational message by using recycled materials. Upcycling is taking discarded materials and repurposing them for a new and better use.

You'll need a plastic blister pack like from a pack of batteries, magic markers, or small toy. Find an image that resonates with you and that fits inside the plastic and find a word or phrase that matches the image. Glue these down to a piece of cardstock or reused cardboard from something like a tissue box. After you glue the transparent plastic on top of the words, wrap decorative paper around the plastic edges to cover it up. Punch a hole on top to hang. Voila! You have a unique piece of art from recycled materials that is fun keep or give as a gift.

I first learned of this process from Rochester, NY artist Martha Schermerhorn.[8] Her pieces are whimsical and full of humor. She calls them *Ikon-a-Pacs*.

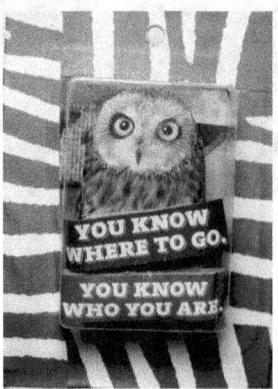

This is one of my upcycled art pieces, *You Know Where To Go.*

---

[8] www.mostlyartistsbooks.com

Color A Mandala

When I was working with adolescent girls in a lock up detention center, I offered my clients copies from my *Coloring Mandalas* book by Susanne Fincher. The girls loved them. They had a lot of time on their hands, as well as a lot of pent up anger and sadness. The simple exercise of coloring a mandala relieved some stress in their young, developing bodies and minds.

If it worked for the girls, why wouldn't it work for you? Get your colored pencils or crayons and start coloring. You can also find ready-to-print blank mandalas on the internet. You'll quickly find yourself in a zone of relaxation.

The word *mandala* comes from the Sanskrit language. It literally means "circle." In Hinduism and Buddhism, mandalas are sacred art and meditational devices meant to produce focus and awareness.

Have you ever seen Tibetan Buddhist monks creating sand mandalas? Colored sand is gracefully and slowly arranged on the ground in the form of a mandala, often with intricately designed concentric circles and vibrant colors. It is beautiful. Once the sand mandala is completed, however, it's destroyed by blowing it away and cleaning it up to symbolize the fleeting and transitory nature of material life.

Photography Phun

Catherine Anderson of Charlotte, North Carolina, eloquently explains the spiritual process of photography in her new book, *The Creative Photographer*:

> *There is magic in the process of making a photograph. For me, it is a way to express beauty, rawness, age, time, and other emotions and feelings that I can't put into words. It is a way of expressing who I am...It almost feels like bottling time. When I take a photograph that speaks to me on this deep level, I can only describe it as a spiritual experience.*
>
> *The creative process of photography allows me to be fully present, to see the beauty that surrounds me, and to feel gratitude for the amazing world I live in. It allows me to recognize the miraculous in everyday moments. These are considerable gifts.*
>
> *...Photography is like visual journaling, and what we are drawn to photograph can speak to us in a symbolic way. We all see the same*

thing, but we see it differently, and our images show others how we see the world... There is no competition. There is no rush. Use your camera as a way to slow down and see with your eyes wide open, to see with your heart.

After reading her words, are you moved to use your camera for self-expression? I sure am. My latest photography kick is with my iPhone using the application called Instagram. It's a fun way to use technology to bottle time. The Instagram community is active and talented too. View photos from around the world in real time.

Another phun photography idea is to take daily snapshots of yourself. Why? For some it's simply interesting to see changes over time. For others it's a healing process for self-hate issues and learning to love oneself. No matter why these folks do it, photography is the medium they choose. How long do you have to do it? That's up to you. A couple weeks, months or years. There are online sites you can use to keep you motivated, which means you'd use your computer's camera or a digital camera, and then upload your photos. Daily self-portrait snapshots can be taken with a Polaroid camera to get an instant print and hang the collection on the wall or store them in a box.

www.dailymugshot.com allows you to feed into your Twitter or

Facebook account

www.flickaday.com

www.flickr.com has daily self-portrait groups and a couple weekly groups like Self-Portrait Thursdays

Mixed Media using an Altoid Tin Box

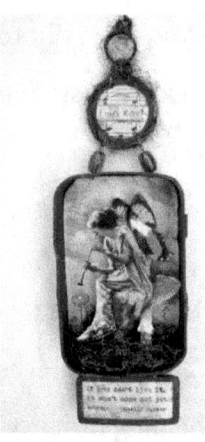

Musical Fairy Muse – Live It

by www.etsy.com/shop/shadesoflimonium

Remember creating dioramas in school? Altered Altoid tin boxes are a little like those. There are no rules or suggestions. Just start gluing! Wouldn't these been fun gifts? Or fun to decorate and put gifts inside?

The empty box beckons to be filled with momentos, images, or words. It's possible to organize, design, and complete this craft project in one sitting. If you have made one, I would love to see it! Please post it to this book's Facebook Forum page www.facebook.com/NOWnoordinarywoman

CHAPTER 6

OTHER CREATIVE OUTLETS

More creative stuff to do? Why, YES! I often hear in my workshops and from women I meet, "Well, I'm just not creative." I simply don't believe it. Here are more ideas for you to express yourself. Thereby, you will engage in self-care, learn something about yourself, and if your Inner Critique is turned off and you're enjoying the process, you'll also raise your positive vibration.

Get Typing

Words matter. And you know it. You have a notebook full of poems or ideas for children's books. Or perhaps you have an outline for an exciting novel. Or maybe there's a memoir inside you waiting to come out, with hopes to share your challenges and knowledge with others. FanStory and Women on Writing can help get your fingers typing.

FanStory is a website that allows you to you submit your story or poem and get unbiased feedback. The site also hosts writing contests such as 500 word flash fiction, haiku, horror stories, and more.

www.fanstory.com

Women on Writing is a comprehensive website for authors, editors, literary agents, publishers, and readers. The site's resources include interviews, articles, and classes. They also have contests.

www.wow-womenonwriting.com

Get Your Squidoo On

Squidoo. Pronounced like "squid-due." Funny word, right? The title lends itself to the whole gestalt of the website. Squidoo is fun, easy to navigate, and full of useful information. You've lived enough years to gather information and develop tastes and opinions. You know what you *know*. Now share your knowledge with others on Squidoo. Why? Because others will benefit from your personal stories and knowledge. Besides informing others, here's a chance to dip your toe in the online publishing pool. Test your writing skills by joining this free online community. Writing a simple Squidoo one pager is a valuable exercise for you at any time, but it's particularly useful before you create a website or a full blog.

It's a fun environment with Squidoo's points and trophies. A few of my pages from years ago are *What are Expressive Arts Therapy and Creative Arts Therapy?*, *Top 25 Abstract Paintings (by artists who are alive and kicking),* and *My Toddler's Favorite 12 Books.* Even though I wrote these pages many years ago, I still get messages about them by people wanting to know more. In addition, Squidoo ranks high with SEOs (search engine optimizations), so if you already have a website and business, having a Squidoo page may help increase traffic for you.

What should you write about? Anything. Seriously, anything. Whatever jazzes you. It's a simply way to exercise your writing itch. Do you have a special way you pick your basketball teams for March Madness? Do you love your neighborhood or hometown? Are there stacks of romance novels in your home? After writing a Squidoo page about your 16 favorite books, maybe it's time to try your hand at writing your own novel or creating a website that reviews romance novels written by women. Can you really make a living reviewing books? Yep. Check out www.bookslut.com for inspiration. This particular site receives about 6,500 unique visitors per day.

An alternative to Squidoo is Hubpages.

Rock Out At Ladies Rock Camp

That's right, Ladies Rock Camp! It's a weekend camp for women with or without any prior musical knowledge to rock out. The first time I heard about this was in *Bust Magazine* and I thought it was the coolest idea. Women of all ages and social backgrounds get together for a weekend and form real bands. The instrument choices are usually drums, bass, lead guitar, or vocals. During these few days of camp, the women write an original song, learn their instrument of choice, practice, and then perform their songs live. It gets even cooler! The fee for the weekend goes towards funding the Girls' Rock Program, which empowers the next generation. There are LRCs in Brooklyn, Portland, OR, Oakland, Philadelphia, Austin, Chicago, Boston, and Los Angeles. Attending a LRC has been on my bucket list and on my vision boards for a couple of years now. Maybe I'll see you at LRC and we'll be in band together?

Be a Recording Artist! Mix Your Own Songs and Beats

You've seen images of music studios where executives sit behind a big soundboard with a bunch of dials and knobs. They're job is to come up with new beats, rhythms, and songs. I think that would be an awesome career! Now you can try your hand at mixing up a new sound online at Soundation. The website is www.soundation.com/studio and it's free to use. It's so easy to lay down tracks. Just click, grab and let go.

Try layering 125 909 Kick.wav over top of 125 Bass Chop C.wav. Then mix in a little 90 BeatMike.wav and 125 Synth Darknight2.wav. It'll get you grooving!   Also 125 PercArabic is a fun bellydancing clip.

Create an Altar

According to Harriet Tubman Wright[9] of Oakland, CA, *"An altar is a visual and tangible center of focus that grounds, uplifts and transforms energy. Creating your own customized altar will shift your energy and your environment. Align yourself with what's most important in your life, beginning with you, the soul essence of you, and begin anew in your life today."* Harriet is available for in-home consultations or phone consultations.

The process can be done on your own as well. Here are some of my ideas.

What in your life do you want to meditate on or honor? It could be your transition to becoming an empty nester, turning 40, about your business blossoming, or about a relationship. There are no rules. This is a very personal process.

The first step is to decide where you want your home altar – inside, outside, bedroom, living room? Next, decide where in the room feels like a good place to set up. Would it be best on a credenza, table, shelf, floor, window sill, amongst plants, or in a closet? You can mark off a space using a cloth or a piece of fabric.

---

[9] www.thewrightresort.com

Gather photos, images, objects, or materials from nature that represents whatever you want to honor. Then arrange all the items in a way that comforts you.

Check in with your altar daily or even twice a day, when you awake and before you go to sleep. Checking in means something different for everyone. You could do a chant, sing a song, read a poem or a verse. Or you could simply stand in silence.

Kickstarter Fun

Do you have a creative idea that you are so passionate about launching but don't have the funds to do it? Do you have a music cd you've been wishing to produce? Do you have a comic book series just waiting to get printed? How long has that fiction manuscript been sitting on your shelf? At Kickstarter, www.kickstarter.com, you can post your idea, offer incentives, and try to get funding. Say you're a photographer wanting to do an exhibit on flowers growing next to graffiti but you need the funds for the supplies, income, and marketing. After crunching the numbers, $800 is needed for the exhibit. To entice people to pledge to your exhibit idea, you can offer incentives. For example, if someone pledges $5 to your project, you'll send them a small digital copy of one of your photos. If someone pledges $50, you'll send them an 8x10 print of their choice.

If you're more of an arts appreciator, you can still enjoy Kickstarter. As a supporter, you can pledge any amount of money to help compelling creative projects come to life. Some projects accept donations as small as $2. Imagine the excitement and gratitude someone would feel if you, a complete stranger, funded their dream! Now that's an awesome random act of kindness.

Feng Shui Your Bedroom

Feng Shui is a system that helps improve the Qi (energy) of your home and to create an atmosphere of harmony and peace.

Master Louisa Ong-Lee of Feng Shui 8[10] gives consultations for homes and businesses. She worked on the Marina Bay Sands Integrated Resort in Singapore and also on other multi-million dollar projects. Here's a tip she gives for your bedroom: "*In the bedroom, always display items in pairs, for example, a pair of birds, a pair of giraffes, a pair of rabbits, etc. This will symbolically attract romance or enhance an existing marriage.*"

The pair in my bedroom are minimal sketches of a nude man and a nude woman that my mother-in-law, Jill Cerulli[11], quickly sketched in one of her drawing classes. Now is that cool or just weird to have

---

[10] www.fengshui8998.com
[11] www.jillcerulli.com

sketched nudes in your bedroom that your mother-in-law drew?

Are you down with P.O.D.?

Get creative by printing a set of your travel photographs as greeting cards for yourself or to give as gifts. Decorate a mug with your baby's face. Create a funny t-shirt. You can do all this and more very simply. P.O.D. = Print on Demand, and these websites offer print on demand services: Zazzle, Café Press, and Red Bubble. You do not need to be a graphic designer or tech savvy to make products for reasonable prices. If you really enjoy creating in this way, you can take your art and ideas one step further and open an online shop on each of these websites and sell your products.

On the other hand, if you're looking for unique gifts, peruse these sites. You won't find these items at the mall or in a catalog. In addition, you'll be supporting small business owners.

CHAPTER 7

LET THE GOOD TIMES ROLL

All work and no play isn't good for anyone! Have fun with these creative living ideas!

Hit The Road

There is nothing like traveling and experiencing fresh sights, sounds, foods, and people. I've always been a gadabout and continue to live with wanderlust. Many of my friends and acquaintances are of the same ilk. One buddy shared these house exchange websites that he and his family, which include young children, use to travel. A house exchange provides a unique travel experience and saves money. There are different options for exchange. One option is to have an even exchange, meaning you go to someone's house at the same time they stay at your house. Most of the sites are free to join. Read the testimonials and use common sense when considering a house exchange.

www.hospitalityclub.org

www.homeexchange.com

www.homeforexchange.com

www.sabbaticalhomes.com – I have personal experience with this one since my husband is in the academic world. Great resource.

Now my niece, who is in her twenties, educated me about www.CouchSurfing.org. This is another alternative way to travel and meet people.   The ethos is simple; you sleep on people's couches when you travel, hence the name. After signing up for free, you look for people in your destination city who have a spare couch, bed, or room and you send them a message. If you're open-minded and have a spare couch, bed, or guest room, then you list your home as available for travelers on the site.

I like how all these sites instill a sense of community on a macro level while the connections happen on a micro level...one spare couch or bed at a time.

Postcard Penpal Fun

So maybe you're not ready to have someone sleeping on your coach or you won't be exchanging houses with anyone in Argentina next year. But that doesn't mean you can't "see" the world and meet new folks. Check out www.postcrossing.com. After registering for free, you'll receive random names from around the world to which you send a postcard. Eventually, you'll receive random, surprise postcards from around the world as well. It's not a one-to-one exchange. You don't know from which country your cards will come. If you have children or teenagers, joining this website is a great opportunity to discuss geography and history with them. Or if you homeschool, maybe this could be part of your social studies curriculum. This activity teaches that the world is a big but kind place. I have a huge map on a wall with yarn connecting the received postcards to the countries from which they came. My youngster gets very excited when a new postcard arrives in the mail and we run to the postcard wall to search for the country. It's fun to hear a preschooler say "Belarus!," "Malaysia!," and "The Netherlands!" Even if I didn't have a child, I know I would still be a member and also have the postcard wall. It's that much fun!

Find New Buddies

Creative living includes meeting new people! One way is through www.MeetUp.com. When I moved again I didn't know anyone in the new city nor did I know anything about the area. Consequently, I checked out Meetup and joined a brunch club. I don't go any longer but I did meet a bunch of nice people and it was great to try new restaurants in the area. There are Meetups for EVERYTHING – play bridge, eat and discuss raw food diet, go motorcycle riding, see international movies, mothers' groups, financial planning for beginners, swing dancing, hiking, sushi lovers, book clubs, coffee shop gatherings, small dog groups, and many, many more. Check it out to find folks who have interests similar to your own in your area.

Share Your Expertise on HARO

Creative living is about trying new things and this idea is pretty new for most readers. Have you ever been the subject of a magazine article? It could be fun being interviewed and sharing your story. Have you ever wondered how people get interviewed for magazines, news, political shows, and talk shows? Chances are these people pitched their expertise to reporters. HARO (Help A Reporter Out) is one resource writers use to find people to fill their stories.[12] It's a chance for you to share your knowledge and experience. Writers, reporters, producers, and bloggers are looking for fresh angles daily. After you register with the site, you'll receive daily emails listing story ideas and the kinds of people needed to interview and/or share their experience. There are close to 30,000 journalists and over 100,000 sources registered with HARO.

Music To Your Ears

If you're tired of the song rotation on Top 40 radio, then you'll sing to the mountaintops with these alternatives.

---

[12] www.helpareporter.com

Epitonic is an online source for independent music which allows songs to be downloaded for free and legally! Lately, I've been digging the "Lo-Fi" and "Drum and Bass" genres. Go mining for some new grooves!

Cd Baby and ReverbNation honors indie music-makers, folks who blaze their own trails by producing their own music. These musicians aren't waiting to be picked up by major labels to live their passions. Enjoy the sounds of up-and-comers from around the globe. Every musical genre is available: hip hop, world, rock, alternative, new age, avant garde, children, and also spoken word.

Lastfm and Pandora Radio are two streaming music websites that "predict" songs for you by evaluating your song choices. Just sit back and let the computer do the song mining for you.

Random Act of Kindness with Books (like this one!)

Have you walked by an expired meter in front of a stranger's car and put a coin into it because you saw the meter maid approaching? Or have you ever mailed a greeting card to someone telling them you were thinking of them? Or do you ever hold the door for someone behind you? These are random acts of kindness (RAK) and they make people feel good. RAKs are little doses of positivity that society needs to balance all of the unpleasantness in life.

Here's one way to perform a RAK with books:

Why not brighten someone's day with a surprise book? Bookcrossing is an online community devoted to this endeavor. The website can be a little confusing but the basic premise is this: You have a book you want to release into the world. You may or may not have read it. Whatever the case, you want it out there. Go to www.bookcrossing.com and register the book to get a Bookcrossing identification number for the book. This number gets written in the book with instructions. Then you give this book to someone you know. Or you can leave it in a public place, like a park bench, decorated (to bring attention to it) with an explanation of what's going on. The hope is that the finder/receiver will be elated, go to the website, enter in the identification number, write a quick post about where they found it, and say whether or not they liked the book and why. Then they, too, will do the same thing and pass the book on.

There are so many variables that could make this operation a success or not. The website states that only about 20% of the registered books get found. But I think it's still a really cool concept.

Of course, you don't need to be part of Bookcrossing to do this

RAK. You can leave or give a surprise book to whomever and whenever. You can use something other than books too.

I encountered a RAK last spring. I found a Ziploc bag with a disposable camera in my library's hallway. On the way to the lost and found, a brightly colored note attached to the bag caught my attention. The note explained it was a project for a photography student at a local college. It asked the finder to take photos and then leave the camera somewhere for another community participant. The student requested the disposable camera be mailed back to her dorm mailbox after all the photos were taken. I snapped a couple photos and then left it on a bench along a frequented walking path. The next day, the baggie with the camera was gone. I hoped the undergraduate's photography project continued and I was glad to be part of it. It was a triple RAK – I shot a few photos for the young woman's class assignment, she gave me a surprise and chance to photograph local images that are dear to me, and I got to leave it for someone else to experience it.

Healthy Living

Take care of your body, it's the only place you have to live.
Jim Rohn

We're so busy; we ignore it and only give it frustrated attention when something is out of whack. We are caregivers and forget about ourselves. Not any more, your health is non-negotiable. Take care of yourself.

Chapter 8 Your Body, discusses a variety of physical issues that can be addressed with alternative and holistic answers. Chapter 9 What's Going In? brings awareness to what is actually going in your mouth. Chapter 10 You Are So Beautiful, looks at ways to beautify but in a healthy living kind of way. Chapter 11 Keep The Crazies In Check: Your Emotional and Mental Health, covers the other side of healthy living – the health of your mind and spirit.

CHAPTER 8

YOUR BODY

Thermal Imaging for Breast Cancer, An Alternative

Mammograms expose the body to radiation. Thermal Imaging or thermography is an alternative diagnostic tool without the radiation of standard mammograms. Instead, in thermal imaging your body is scanned for heat and inflammation to detect an issue or abnormality. It's non-invasive, painless, there's no body contact, and it's FDA approved. Your insurance may or may not cover the cost of a session. Depending on your insurance coverage, Flex Spending and Health Savings Accounts may be used for this session. Call your insurance carrier for details.

Thermal imaging can be used for other health screenings as well, such as unexplained pain, arthritis, digestive disorders, and fibromyalgia.

Vitamin D3 – Are you Deficient?

There's been a lot of talk over the years suggesting that women are deficient in vitamin D3. It's in the news and in magazines.

According to the Vitamin D Council:

> *Current research has implicated vitamin D deficiency as a major factor in the pathology of at least 17 varieties of cancer as well as heart disease, stroke, hypertension, autoimmune diseases, diabetes, depression, chronic pain, osteoarthritis, osteoporosis, muscle weakness, muscle wasting, birth defects, periodontal disease, and more.*
>
> *Vitamin D's influence on key biological functions vital to one's health and well-being mandates that vitamin D no longer be ignored by the health care industry nor by individuals striving to achieve and maintain a greater state of health.* [13]

A blood test given by your doctor can check for vitamin D3 deficiency. Or a home test can be bought on the internet depending on which country you reside and if in the USA, depending on which state you're located. After speaking with your doctor, vitamin D3 supplements can be purchased as liquid drops, chews, or pills.

---

[13] www.vitamindcouncil.org

Adrenal Fatigue – The Busy Woman's Concern

Our small adrenal glands sit on top of our kidneys. They're responsible for many functions including producing estrogen, testosterone, progesterone, and cortisol. According to Dr. Leila Kirdani of The Centre for Optimum Health in Rochester, NY, adrenal fatigue comes from prolonged stress or after a major stressor such as surgery, car accident, or divorce. She states that *"Our bodies were built for danger, not for chronic stress. We were designed to stay alive in the face of mortal danger. When the tiger jumps out of the bush at us, our cortisol (fight or flight hormone) immediately increases. This causes an increase in blood sugar, so our muscles and brain have fuel to run from the tiger...In the 21st century we are facing 'tigers' all the time. Our tigers today are childhood trauma, relationships, finances, time, job stress, car accidents, and a toxic environment. Chronically increased blood sugar leads to belly fat and eventually diabetes. Chronically increased inflammation leads to numerous medical problems including hypertension, asthma, allergies, arthritis, obesity, muscle and joint pain."*

Do you feel exhausted? Do you get sick often? Are you irritable? Do you crave sugar or caffeine? If you answer yes to any of these questions, talk with your doctor or alternative health care professional about the possibility of adrenal fatigue. They may test your saliva or do a hair analysis. If you do have adrenal fatigue, diet and nutrition are important factors to review, as are supplements and stress relieving activities.

Two Belly Rubs for Maximum Health Benefits

Irritable Bowel Syndrome, constipation, diarrhea, fertility problems, endometriosis, and ulcers are just a few problems we have in our belly region. Instead of, or in addition to, medication, the following two massages may bring you relief.

Maya Abdominal Massage (also called The Arvigo Techniques of Maya Abdominal Therapy) is a massage for women and men focusing on the area from below your ribs down to your pubic bone out to the sides of your body. This explanation is from the website: *"The techniques work to bring about correct position of organs that have shifted and now restrict the flow of blood, lymph, nerve & chi energy. In short the Arvigo Techniques seek to restore the body to its natural balance."*[14] Most massages skip the abdomen, which is odd because so many people hold tension in their gut. I had a session or two in my late 20s for irregular menstrual cycles and it helped.

Chi Nei Tsang (CNT) is another form of abdominal "massage." In CNT, the focus is on working the energy of the internal organs. CNT

---

[14] www.arvigotherapy.com

detoxifies a person both physically and emotionally. Intestinal problems can stem from emotional issues and during a CNT session emotional release can happen. If you're ever in Oakland, CA book an appointment with the CNT Institute's Director Gilles Marin. It's a unique healing experience. Or you could find a practitioner near you from a listing on their website[15].

Earthing and EMFs

You can't see it, smell, or taste it but it's there.

Electropollution, radiation outputs, and EMFs (electromagnetic fields) are controversial issues these days. There is research claiming one thing and then more research debunking it. Even though I try to educate myself, I still find theories a little confusing since I'm neither an electrician, physicist, nor electrical engineer.

But one thing is for sure, the sheer amount of electronic gadgets in our houses have increased over the years. We have cell phones, iPhones, iPads, laptops and notebook computers. Many people are surrounded by these items all day long. We also have our appliances, cordless phones, microwave ovens, cell phone towers, televisions, power lines and wi-fi/wireless connections. At places of businesses, like hospitals, there's even more equipment to

---

[15] www.chineitsang.com

consider.

In Dr. Samuel Milham's book, *Dirty Electricity: Electrification and the Diseases of Civilization,* he states "We are an electrochemical soup at the cellular and organ level...We evolved in a complex EMF environment with an interplay of natural terrestrial and extra-terrestrial EMF sources from solar activity, cosmic rays, and geomagnetic activity. I believe that our evolutionary balance, developed over the millennia, has been severely disturbed and disrupted by man-made EMFs." His book goes on to describe case study after case study of the diseases caused by electromagnetic fields and radio frequency radiation from cell phones and cellular phone towers, wi-fi, and personal electronic equipment, including leukemia, male breast cancer, and diabetes.

The Radiation Research Trust campaign "Save the Male" is warning men not to carry their mobile phones in their trouser pockets as it can affect their fertility.[16] The evidence strongly suggests that sperm is damaged significantly (lower sperm counts and reduced sperm motility) from cell phone radiation. I wonder why there's no research for females carrying their phones in their pockets. Is it because women usually carry a purse or because our ovaries and eggs aren't as susceptible as sperm? Also the website warns: "Just 30 minutes a day on a phone increases your chance of

---

[16] www.radiationresearch.org

getting brain cancer by 40%. If you use a mobile [phone] for 10 years or more you are 290% more likely to get brain tumors and cancer." Maybe it's time to consider those wire microphones to plug into the mobile phone? Or use a landline when possible?

In the State of Maine, a bill was created called the Children's Wireless Protection Act, which would require that cell phones are sold with this warning label:

> WARNING, THIS DEVICE EMITS
> ELECTROMAGNETIC RADIATION, EXPOSURE TO
> WHICH MAY CAUSE BRAIN CANCER. USERS,
> ESPECIALLY CHILDREN AND PREGNANT
> WOMEN, SHOULD KEEP THIS DEVICE AWAY
> FROM THE HEAD AND BODY.

Schools are taking matters into their own hands and removing or not installing wi-fi in their building so as not to expose children and teachers to low level microwave radiation all day long for years at a time. St. Vincent Euphrasia Elementary, a school in southern Ontario, Canada has banned and turned off their wi-fi due to health concerns, stating that it was an unnecessary risk. All of their computers are now plugged in with hardwires.

For more information about EFTs and electropollution, visit

Microwave News at www.microwavenews.com. They've been around for 30 years reporting on the dangers of EMFs and radiation to our health and environment. Also, Mobile Wise is a website geared toward educating teens on potential health risks when using their cell phones.[17]

So what can you do? Again, there's a lot of conflicting information out there. What's necessary to protect yourself and what is effective is still up in the air as far as I can tell. But the following are a few ideas.

First, check out Ann Louise Gittleman's book, *Zapped: Why Your Cell Phone Shouldn't Be Your Alarm Clock and 1,268 Ways to Outsmart the Hazards of Electronic Pollution.* This book is full of useful tips that are understandable and can be executed.

In addition, meters are available to measure radiation and harmful electromagnetic outputs in your life. There are also ways to shield yourself. EMF shielding clothing and bed canopies are possible solutions. Another option is to literally ground yourself as often as possible. Grounding is also called earthing.

Simply put, grounding/earthing is having direct contact with the Earth. There has been substantial research on the positive effects of walking barefoot in grass, sand, dirt, cement or anywhere that

---

[17] www.mobilewise.org

puts you in direct contact with the Earth. Walking, sitting, or playing barefoot on the Earth reconnects your body to the natural electrical field from the Earth, thus bringing your body's internal electrical state into balance. People who are grounded feel more relaxed. But, significantly, this grounding can also help with a multitude of other health issues, such as better sleep, menstrual and hormone balance, and pain reduction.

For more information, refer to the book *Earthing: The Most Important Health Discovery Ever?* by Clinton Ober, Dr. Stephen Sinatra, and Martin Zucker which goes into great detail about why earthing works.

So now you're thinking you want to try this earthing/grounding stuff but it's cold outside or you can't leave your office? When walking outside isn't possible, you can still be connected to the Earth inside your house or office via the ground port in an electrical wall outlet. In the USA outlets accept three-pronged plugs; the small circle hole is the ground port. Check the wiring first using an inexpensive electrical outlet tester to see if it's grounded. There are body bands, bedsheets, mousepads, and foot mats specially made with a grounding cord that plugs into the ground port of the electrical outlet, thus, connecting you to the Earth.

I'm not endorsing any of these products or websites; simply sharing information. I do have a mousepad that is sometimes use as a foot pad as well.

Clint Ober's Earthing Institute
www.earthinginstitute.net

Dr. Anne Louise's website
www.unikeyhealth.com

David Avocado Wolfe's website
www.earthingyou.com

Xenoestrogens and Xena The Warrior Princess Are Not Related

Xenoestrogens are estrogen-like compounds that interfere with normal hormone function and have been linked to breast cancer. The Breast Cancer Fund's report, *State of the Evidence: The Connection between Breast Cancer and the Environment*, has a list of where xenoestrogens come from, including tobacco smoke and parabens found in many shampoos, body lotions, and moisturizers.[18] Styrofoam also contains xenoestrogen Bisephenol-A (BPA), and when it's heated it can leach into your food or drink. Think about how many hot cups of coffee are consumed in Styrofoam cups.

---

[18] www.breastcancerfund.org

Dr. Elizabeth Smith[19] suggests these ways to avoid xenoestrogens:

1. Use glass or ceramics whenever possible to store food and water. Heat up your food using a glass or ceramic bowl covered with dish. When plastic is heated, it diffuses very rapidly into food.

2. Use a simple detergent with less chemicals; Nature Clean is a good choice for both laundry detergent and dish washing detergent.

3. Simple Soap is a safe choice for shampoo and a body soap.

4. Use natural pest control not pesticides.

5. Avoid Synthetic Chemicals - Healthy Living in a Toxic World by Cynthia Fincher PhD. is a good place to start.

6. Don't use herbicides; use a cup of salt in a gallon of vinegar.

7. Buy hormone free meats to eat.

8. Buy "Organic" produce, produce grown without pesticides, herbicides or synthetic fertilizer or hormones.

9. Use Condoms without spermicide for Birth control instead of Birth Control Pills. Use Natural Progesterone instead of HRT.

10. The vast majority of skin lotions and creams use parabens as a preservative. Avoid them at all costs. Instead apply a vegetable oil right after a shower to hydrate the skin and

---

[19] http://www.fibrocystic.com/xeno.htm

lock in the moisture.

Epigenetics – Why You Need to Know

Every cell in your body has the same DNA, the same set of genes. The DNA within a single cell would be more than a yard-long if stretched out. How does nature fit this long stretch of DNA into the nucleus of a single cell? By winding the DNA around a core, like thread around a spool. When the DNA is tightly wrapped around the core it is not available to be turned on. Nature has developed means of "loosening" particular stretches of tightly wrapped DNA, however, so that it becomes available to be turned on. The field of study that is concerned with making DNA (genes) available to be turned on is called epigenetics. Epigenetics is a new field and there is still much to be learned.

Why should you care about epigenetic and molecular biology? Because these subfields of biology not only determine what parts of our cellular makeup control whether a cell turns into skin, muscle, bone or brain, they also also determine how the cell behaves (or does not behave) once it is formed. In a laboratory study of identical twins—i.e., two people with the same DNA—Professor Paul Coleman, Senior Scientist and Lab Head of Banner Sun Health Research Institute in Arizona has shown that exposure to pesticides can change a person's epigenetic makeup, so that one of a pair of identical twins can experience brain deterioration and get Alzheimer's disease while the other did not. Other studies have shown that the food you eat can control aspects of epigenetics that determine whether diseases such as cancer, hypertension, and diabetes can develop. Studies from several laboratories, most notably that of Professor JD Sweatt at the University of Alabama, have shown that epigenetics play a powerful role in learning and memory. What's more, emerging evidence tells us that some effects of epigenetics can be passed from one generation to the next.

Epigenetics may be the key to healing and prevention in the future. Keep your eyes and ears open for new research findings because epigenetics may be relevant to you or someone you love.

Kiss Your Dentist Goodbye, Sort of

Dr. Ellie Phillips, author of *Kiss Your Dentist Goodbye: A Do It Yourself Mouth Care System for Healthy, Clean Gums and Teeth*, claims to have the ideal strategy for taking care of your pearly whites, thus eliminating or reducing your need to visit to the dentist.[20] Her strategy includes familiar products like Crest toothpaste, Listerine, and ACT® Anticavity Flouride and non-familiar items like Closys and Xylitol.

---

[20] www.zelliescleanwhiteteeth.com

The system has three steps:

Step 1: Clean and Brush - rinse with Closys then brush with Crest toothpaste

Step 2: Freshen – rinse with Listerine

Step 3: Protect – Rinse with ACT Fluoride

Also use Xylitol as a sweetener, gum, or mint.

A bit on Xylitol from her website:

> *Xylitol is a delicious weapon in the fight against dental disease. It looks and tastes like sugar but has 40% fewer calories. When xylitol dissolves in your mouth, it makes a sweet sugary solution that is alkaline, the opposite of damaging acidic. Xylitol is diabetic friendly. Xylitol is organic and all natural — found in the fibers of fruits and vegetables like corn, berries and mushrooms, and the wood of trees like the birch. It is even produced naturally in small amounts by our bodies.*

Dr. Ellie makes gum and mints from Xylitol. For details on Dr. Ellie's system, do an online search for "NEWZelliesCompleteMouthcareSystem.pdf"

Here's another alternative to your dental care. It's a radical change from what you have been taught about taking care of your teeth. Nadine Artemis of Living Libations[21] has created a system of self-dentistry. At the heart of her system is a product called Healthy Gum Drops, which is a liquid created from essential oils of seabuckthorn berry, rose, oregano, peppermint, cinnamon, clove, tea tree, and thyme linalool. Nadine claims that the combination of these oils serves as anti-bacterial nourishment for the gums, teeth and saliva; it also takes care of plaque, bleeding and receding gums, tooth sensitivity and decay. The reviews of Healthy Gum Drops have been very positive. People seem to really enjoy brushing their teeth with Nadine's botanical blend because of the truly clean refreshing feeling it offers, and many folks claim to have had better visits to the dentist as a result of using Healthy Gum Drops.

I just ordered my own Healthy Gum Drops and want to experience this alternative to toothpaste. I once tried tooth soap as an alternative to toothpaste and wasn't a fan. I'm curious to see if Healthy Gum Drops are a more palatable option.

Speaking of oils and dental care, I once treated a mild toothache with Thieves Oil. Thieves Oil is made of clove, lemon, cinnamon bark, eucalyptus, and rosemary. I added a diluted drop to an ear cleaner (to some, a cotton bud) and placed it on top of the tooth

---

[21] www.livinglibations.com

and lightly bit down for a minute. The pain vanished quickly and hasn't returned. As with anything in this book, please seek professional health advice before trying anything new.

BIG Health Benefits From a Little of This Oil

Oil of oregano is an herbal oil used for a spat of different health concerns; it is not a cooking oil. It comes in a bottle with a dropper or in capsules. Herbalists and others claim that it fights bacteria, fungus, microbes, candida, staph infections, and yeast overgrowth. Again, with any new herb or vitamin or anything, please consult a professional before using. Oil of oregano has been known to reduce iron levels and should not be taken during pregnancy. Feel a cold coming on? Oil of oregano may help combat the germs and shorten the duration of your cold.

I take it when I start to feel sick or when someone in my house is sick. If I take this powerful oil for a few days or more, I also take a probiotic. In the morning I'll take the probiotic and at night I'll take the Oil of Oregano. I do this to keep the intestinal flora healthy.

CHAPTER 9

WHAT'S GOING IN?

How aware are you when it comes to the food and drinks entering your body? Do you consider the healthy benefits you're ingesting, or lack thereof? These tips can help you be mindful of your nutrition.

Fake Meats

Fake meats are typically a staple in the vegetarian diet or in the diet of someone whose doctor instructed them to cut out fried and unhealthy foods. But are they really healthy for you? The jury is out on this one.

Sheri Oppenheimer, Certified Holistic Health Counselor and Co-Founder of The 100 Women Project[22] shared this with me:

> *Eating as close to the source as possible is always the best option. Many fake meat products are made with soy, which, in its natural form, is an excellent source of nutrition*

---

[22] www.100womenproject.com

that many cultures have relied on for centuries for its nutritive benefits. However, many processed soy products contain unhealthy fats and compounds that can be detrimental to our health. Although they are processed, fake meats are still a great alternative to fast food burgers.

Fake meats are high in sodium and also usually made of wheat gluten. If you have a sensitivity to gluten, please read the ingredients. Like many things in life, eating fake meats *in moderation* may be the best option. But what does "in moderation" mean? That's a question for your doctor, nutritionist, or holistic health counselor.

Healthy Pots and Pans

Non-stick coated pans are health hazards because they leach chemicals into food at high temperatures. Leaching chemicals are bad for our bodies since they can cause many health problems like cancer, infertility, and more. There are reports of pet birds dying due to the hazardous fumes produced from heating non-stick pans coated in Teflon.[23] So, if this stuff is hurting birds what is it doing to us?

---

[23] http://www.ewg.org/reports/toxicteflon

The alternatives to consider for your cooking needs include stainless steel, enamel cast iron, and ceramic. Le Creuset is one company that makes enamel cast iron cookware. Another option is Cusinart's eco-friendly line called Green Gourmet and is petroleum-free, PTFE/PFOA-free. PTFE is polytetrafluoroethylene and PFOA is perfluorooctanoic acid and both are synthetics. Cuisanart's Green Gourmet frying pan is made of Ceramica™ instad. But neither the packaging nor the website explains what Ceramica™ is or what the raw materials are.

Celtic Sea Salt and Himalayan Salt – Small Change, Big Benefits

Because regular table salt is processed and chemically treated, many valuable minerals are removed in its production. Unrefined sea salt and Celtic sea salt, on the other hand, are healthier because they aren't chemically treated. Iodine, iron, calcium, magnesium, manganese, potassium and zinc are found in unrefined sea salts and Celtic sea salt. The small, simple switch from regular table salt to sea salt is healthier for you and your family.

Himalayan salt comes from the salt range in the Himalayan Mountains and is also free of chemical processing. Salt lamps, made from Himalayan salt, oxygenate and purify the air. *Nature also renews us because living things resonate at a frequency supported in an organic environment—and this can be disrupted by*

EMFs (Electromagnetic Fields) from mobile phones, computers and electrical devices. Pure crystal salt has harnessed the earth's energy for eons and resonates at a frequency that combats EMF pollution."[24] For more info on EMFs, go to Chapter 8 in this book.

Quinoa vs Rice

White rice has very little nutritional value and has a high glycemic index. This means that it causes blood sugar to rise rapidly, promoting the development of blood sugar disorders, diabetes, and weight gain. In addition to all of this, white rice is constipating.[25] Brown rice is healthier because it hasn't had the natural bran removed from it so there's more fiber and vitamins.

Quinoa (pronounced "keen-wah") is an excellent substitution for white rice. It comes in brown and red varieties and has a nutty taste. It's rich in amino acids and protein. In the cookbook *Veganomicon*, Isa Chandra Moskowitz and Terry Hope Romero explain that *"Quinoa is also a complete protein, which has recently made it something of a darling to the vegan community and health-conscious foodies."* I enjoy the taste of it and how easy it is to prepare.

---

[24] http://www.natural-salt-lamps.com/saltcrystallamps.html
[25] http://www.whole-body-detox-diet.com/brown-rice.html

Get Raw with Your Honey and Your Chocolate

Raw foods are unprocessed foods. Therefore raw foods have more nutritional value because the vitamins and minerals have not been burned out by heat or lost in a myriad of other chemicals during manufacturing and processing. There are many (un)cookbooks with tasty recipes for getting more raw foods into your diet. If you're imagining just eating celery sticks and apples, once you do a little research you'll be in for a big yummy surprise.

A few raw (un)cookbooks to get you started:

Ani's Raw Food Kitchen by Ani Phyo
Living Raw Food by Sarma Melngailis
RawEnergy by Stephanie Tourles

When buying honey or chocolate consider choosing raw over their commercial counterparts.

Raw honey hasn't been heated, processed, or strained, thus it contains all the natural nutrients it has right out of the hive. The benefits of raw honey are quickly and widely catching on, and jars can be found in many local grocery stores, not just at farmers' markets or health food stores. Buying local raw honey is a great way to support your local beekeepers, too. Personally, I think it tastes delicious. I was never an avid honey eater until I was introduced to the raw variety.

Raw chocolate, also called raw cacao, comes in powder form or nibs. Here's what's printed on my bag of organic raw cacao powder by Navitas: *"Cacao contains a naturally rich supply of antioxidants and is a good source of dietary fiber. It is also known to be one of the highest dietary sources of magnesium, flavanols, and polyphenols."* Simply put, it's healthier because it's not processed and full of chemicals. I often use it in smoothies. For a treat, I add a tablespoon to a food processor with some walnuts, unprocessed and unsweetened coconut flakes, and chopped dates. After it's all mixed, I form one inch balls and chill in the fridge or freezer.

Oh Ah...Healthy Socca

Socca is a filling thin flatbread that is made of chickpea flour. In France, it's called *socca*. In Italy, it's called *farinata*. Since it's made from chickpea flour it's high in protein, fiber, folic acid, and it's gluten free. Topped with veggies and a little tomato sauce, it's a great alternative to pizza. Chickpea flour is also called gram flour in some stores.

After mixing the chickpea flour and water 1:1, I let it sit on the counter for about 20 minutes. I sauté onions and spinach in olive oil. Then pour a bit of the flour mix into the pan to form a thin pancake and add seasonings. After it cooks on low/medium temperature, I flip it over for about two minutes. Yummm.

The same flour can be used as pakoras batter. 1 cup flour, .75 cup water, tsp of curry powder, dash of salt. Then mix. Then coat your vegetables like cauliflower, onions, squash, mushrooms and deep fry for about 4 minutes. I use coconut oil for the frying. Mmm, good.

Lose the Excuse, It's Time to Juice

Juicing fruits and vegetables provides a bounty of health benefits. Besides taking in vitamins and minerals, having a liquid meal allows the digestive system to take a bit of a break. Imagine the work the liver, stomach, and intestines have to do to break down and digest food. Now imagine the extra work they have to do to digest processed foods.

In Dr. Alejandro Junger's New York Times bestseller book, *Clean,* he incorporates juicing as part of his 21 day detox program because, he writes, "liquid meals are practically ready for absorption, bypassing the need and energy expense of being broken down." As a 40th birthday present to myself, I tried the detox program. My energy increased and I lost about 5 pounds.

Juicing fruits and vegetables requires a countertop juicer. Small citrus hand juicers can't do the necessary work to incorporate juicing into your diet. My favorite juice at the moment is beet-apple-ginger, which I start my day with fairly often. *As a side note*, beet juice can turn your urine to a reddish color so no need to be concerned.

Don't Eat This Food, But Try These Foods

Did you know that you shouldn't eat bananas when you're feeling under the weather because they are mucus-producing? I attended a talk by a naturopath who said that bananas and dairy should be avoided when you're not feeling well, especially if you have a chest or head cold. Good to know this tidbit when cold, flu, and allergy season come around.

On an unrelated note, do you like crunchy foods? Have you experienced the extraordinary crunch of sunchokes and jicama? Sunchokes and jicama can add excitement to your salads. Sunchokes are also called Jerusalem artichokes and both sunchokes and jicama look a bit like a potato. Both are root vegetables and can be eaten raw or cooked. They're crunchy and have a texture like a water chestnut. Both are high in potassium. Cut into small pieces and add to a salad, or cut into thick slices use for dips and crudité.

CHAPTER 10

YOU ARE SO BEAUTIFUL

You are. Just face it. You're be-you-tee-full! These healthy tips will keep ya lookin' good.

Know the Dirty Dozen Before Putting Them On Your Skin

Who would think that beauty and grooming products could adversely affect your health? The repeated use of toxic chemicals, many of which are found in widely used and sold commercial beauty products, can cause problems. Additionally, the accumulation of these chemicals is a serious problem, since many women and men use multiple products per day: soap, shampoo, conditioner, deodorant, nail polish, perfumes, and lotions.

One place to start your research is www.safercosmetics.org and watch the video *The Story of Safe Cosmetic* with Annie Leonard. Annie explains how and why toxic chemicals are in many of our products, including baby products, and what we can do about it. The site also discusses "pinkwashing," which describes companies that advocate for breast cancer awareness but continue to use chemicals that cause cancer. A total contradiction, right?

Also surprising is the allowance of such products to be manufactured. Many of the chemicals that continue to be used in "health" and beauty products in the United States, Canada, and Mexico have been banned in Europe and Central America. But why not in North America?

Keys Soap, a company based in Annapolis, MD, calls the chemicals typically found in shampoo, conditioner, hair coloring, shaving cream, body lotion, makeup, face moisturizer, bath soaps and gels, nail polish and treatments the Dirty Dozen and states, "At Keys, we believe that over 50% of skin disorders are caused by one or more of these chemicals."

1. sodium/ammonium lauryl sulfate (SLS) – alters skin structure, allowing other chemicals to penetrate

2. parabens – may cause skin irritation, rash, dermatitis, or allergic reaction

3. propylene glycol – alters skin structure, skin irritant, allergic reactions

4. phthalates – damage the liver, kidneys, lung

5. petroleum – allergic reactions

6. cocamide DEA/lauramide DEA – may form carcinogenic nitrosamines

7. diazolidinyl urea – impurities linked to cancer or other health problems

8. butyl acetate – repeated exposure causes skin dryness, cracking

9. butylated hydroxytoluene – eye and skin irritant

10. ethyl acetate – eye and skin irritant

11. toluene – potentially cancer causing, liver damage, skin irritant

12. triethanolamine – may form carcinogenic compounds called nitrosamines

Let's do some math. Say you work a full-time job five days a week. That is 260 days per year you work. There are 10 years between the ages of 30 – 39. Therefore, 260 days per year multiplied by 10 years equals 2,600 days of putting makeup and other grooming products on your face and body. If you're using harmful products, that's 2,600 days of this stuff getting into your bloodstream in one decade.

Let's go even further with our math. For those 2,600 days with makeup on, multiply eight hours a day at work (probably longer since you probably don't wash your face the minute you arrive home), that equals 20,800 hours of this stuff sitting on your face, on your lips, in your hair, in your armpits, and on your eyes. That's a lot of time given to these potential harmful products to wreak havoc to one's system.

For more product education, check out Skin Deep, a beauty products database created by Environmental Working Group. They cover baby and children's products, too. www.ewg.org/skindeep

Mung Bean Body Scrub

I learned about using mung beans for skin care when I lived in India for nine months. Mung beans are legumes, thus, full of vitamins and minerals.

Here's what I do (use at your own risk): Grind up a quarter cup of dry mung beans in a coffee grinder or small food processor until it is almost dust. Place in a ceramic or glass container. When ready to use, mix a tablespoon of mung bean grits with a tablespoon or two of olive oil. I then apply it to my skin in a circular motion as a body scrub and rinse. My skin feels soft afterwards.

When I hear about sugar scrubs or salt scrubs, I wonder what exactly are people rubbing into their skin? Sodium, sugar, unhealthy chemicals? This mung bean scrub seems to be a healthier option.

Beyond Tea Tree Oil

Everyone has probably heard about tea tree oil (also called melaleuca) and its health and beauty uses. While it's a useful product for acne and skin care, there are other essential oils worthy of checking out for your beauty regimen. For example, lavender oil, myrrh oil, and helichrysum oil are said to be beneficial to the skin.

The following information is from the Young Living Essential Oils website[26]:

> *Lavender oil - Lavender is an adaptogen, and therefore can assist the body when adapting to stress or imbalances. It is a great aid for relaxing and winding down before bedtime, yet has*

---

[26] www.youngliving.com

balancing properties that can also boost stamina and energy. Therapeutic-grade lavender is highly regarded for skin and beauty. It may be used to soothe and cleanse common cuts, bruises, and skin irritations.

Myrrh (Commipihora myrrha) has a rich, smoky, balsamic aroma that is purifying, restorative, revitalizing, and uplifting... The Arabian people believed it helped wrinkled, chapped, and cracked skin.

Helichrysum is said to work wonders on wounds and bruises but it it's also useful for rosacea, psoriasis, and dark circles under the eyes.

Besides skin care, these oils can be used for managing headaches and muscle pain, for mood enhancers, for illnesses like the common cold, household cleaning, and for first aid. Organica Jane[27] has a "How To Use" guide that's easy to follow and covers how to use essential oils topically, inhaled, and internally. Also a mini reference guide can be found at http://www.yleo-oils.com/mini-guide.htm. Remember to use a carrier oil when applying oils to skin.

---

[27] www.organicajane.com

Cupping out the Cellulite

I think of cellulite as stubborn fat and toxic deposits that need exercise, blood flow, attention, love, and stretching to go away. Also proper nutrition and eating choices will help prevent and remove it.

I remember hearing about expensive cellulite-removing treatments which included massaging and rolling the cellulite to break it up so it goes away.

Now, there's an at-home alternative to these expensive treatments. Cupping therapy involves little suction-like squishy cups that you hold and attach to the stubborn lumps and move around. Thus, massaging the area. That's it. This simple tool and activity claims to break up and separate the celllite. If haven't tried it yet. If you have, please let me know of your results.

To read about the five stages of cellulite, check out http://bellabaci.com/cellulite.

Hair Care, Oh Yeah

Do you wash your hair every day or just about every day? Well, you may be doing it a disservice. Laura Boton, owner of Sine Qua Non, a successful salon that has four locations in Chicago shared this tip with me:

How often should you wash your hair? Washing hair traditionally implies that you use a detergent based shampoo every day to get clean hair. What that does is strips your hair and scalp of its natural oils every day, causing it to produce more oil at the scalp level while the ends remain dry and brittle. In order to restore your hair and scalp's natural PH balance, only shampoo at the most every other day, and if possible for textured and dry hair, just wet down your hair in the morning daily if you need to and only shampoo once or twice a week to preserve your hair's natural oils. For very dry hair you should try to use a low detergent level shampoo if you shampoo more than once a week. Some of these are called surfactant free.

Less is more. Keep your locks beautiful by not over-washing it.

Yoga and Toning for Your Face

When I was in my 20s, I bought my mother a book for her birthday called *Facercise: Take Ten Years Off your Face in Just Minutes* a Day by Carol Maggio. The gift was to be a gag about her birthday but also to help her age gracefully. Carol Maggio claims to have a proven method of toning the facial muscles, which aid in keeping a youthful appearance sans injections. The book has 14 exercises that target from the forehead down to the lips to soften lines and get rid of sagging. The Forehead Lift is my fave.

Also I'm not sure where I heard this before but a very easy facial toning exercise is to pretend you're blowing out a candle slowly. I think you're supposed to repeat this until you feel "the burn." Yes, your face will get tired! Great to do while driving, at your desk, or while watching a movie.

Search online for an image of the muscles in your face. The exercises will make more sense when you can see the targeted muscles.

One Product That Can Moisturize Your Hair, Body, and Face. Oh, You Can Eat It Too!

Any guesses? Here's a hint: tropical.

No, not bananas. It's coconut oil! This wonderful gift from the tropics has many uses and it's beneficial for your skin because it's antimicrobial and an antioxidant. I buy unrefined organic coconut oil from the health food store. Unrefined means it's raw, not processed, no added chemicals, thus it's pure. It comes in a glass jar and is usually a solid form instead of liquid. But it's not hard; it's mushy and penetrates easily into your skin or hair.

Sometimes, I massage it on my cuticles, heels, and elbows at night. I occasionally use it on my hair as a deep conditioner. I scoop out a tablespoon at a time and apply it to dry hair and scalp. Then wrap my hair in a very light towel and go to sleep. In the morning I wash with shampoo and use conditioner. Or I put it in one hour before taking a shower. My hair feels softer and shinier and I think it helps with split ends. Lately, I've been using as a face moisturizer.

I also found online that that it's used as an eye makeup remover. Women who posted the tip like that it's a natural product used around their eyes and it seems to promote healthier lashes. I've never done this but I assume you apply a little bit to lashes and lids, lightly scrub around and then use a warm, wet wash cloth to remove.

CHAPTER 11

KEEP THE CRAZIES IN CHECK: YOUR MENTAL & EMOTIONAL HEALTH

For whatever reason you're crying, just know that it is normal and actually really good for you to cry because you're releasing pent up emotions. Releasing is essential to mental and physical health. Now, if you find yourself doing this often, then please seek professional help with a traditional talk therapist, energy healer, or expressive arts therapist. Below are some things you can do to keep the "crazies" in check. I say "crazies" with light-heartedness, not with judgment.

EFT and Matrix Reimprinting

A powerful self-help tool that I have utilized is EFT (Emotional Freedom Technique). I'm not alone in using this technique. In February 2011, the free online Tapping Summit hosted by brother and sister team Nick and Jessica Ortner had over 300,000 worldwide participants listening to different EFT experts explain how to use EFT to achieve better relationships, lose weight, gain financial abundance, and alleviate chronic pains.

EFT is a derivative of meridian tapping and has been called psychological acupressure. Eight acupressure/acupuncture points on your head, face, chest, and lateral body are gently tapped with your fingertips while you repeat phrases and verbalize your issue(s). I personally also incorporate acupressure point K1 (kidney 1) located at the center of the ball of the foot. I did this intuitively because my EFT sessions felt incomplete not including the feet. I later learned that this point is for rooting or grounding, which makes sense because whatever issue I'm working on needs to be rooted in my subconscious. Sounds pretty woo-woo, right? Well, it is until you actually try it out for yourself.

These EFT professionals explain and guide you through this simple but powerful process:

Natalie Hill is a wonderful woman from Arizona who's now traveling the world and doing sessions over the Internet and by phone. At the time of this writing she just returned to the USA from living in Thailand. Depending on your issue, Natalie also incorporates Matrix Reimprinting, which helps clear negative blocks from your past so you can move forward. Believe me, you don't know what traumas or Traumas (little "t" for little traumas and big "T" for big Traumas) from your past have formed your current limiting beliefs until you do some work with Natalie. She's helped me become mentally clearer and emotionally lighter, which means I'm more productive and happy.

www.efttappingtechniques.com

Carol Look, a licensed therapist and author, is a wealth of information. Signing up for her e-newsletters allows you to view her archives, which have EFT scripts for a variety of issues like

Feeling Good Instead of Guilty

Fear of Change

When Pain Gets in the Way

Stop Chasing and Start Allowing

www.carollookeft.com

Margaret Lynch has a series of Youtube videos that explain the EFT process, with a special focus on attaining financial happiness.

www.margaretmlynch.com

Pamela Bruner, success coach and author, utilizes EFT to help large and small business owners.

www.makeyoursuccesseasy.com

The Sedona Method

The Sedona Method, created by Hal Dwoskin, is a simple easy-to-learn technique that helps you let go of and release unwanted feelings in the moment. Part of the method focuses on asking yourself three simple questions:

1. Could I let this unwanted emotion go?
2. Would I let it go?
3. When?

Here's how I interpret the method. Say you're at a restaurant celebrating a special occasion with your family and the service isn't as attentive as you'd like it to be. Instead of getting aggravated and allowing this to ruin the night, using this method can help to bring into focus what's important right now, which is quality time with your family. Answering the first question brings the emotion into awareness so you can work with it and not let it control you, per se. Answering the second question gauges the urgency of the situation. Answering the third question prompts you to release the emotion as soon as possible.

1. Could I let this unwanted emotion go? Yes, tonight is about my family.
2. Would I let it go? Yes, it's not that important to use my energy to hold on to it.
3. When? I choose to let it go right now. It won't be beneficial to let it go tonight or tomorrow. I'm letting it go now.

The three questions will be answered according to the intensity level of the situation. For instance, if you just found out your spouse has been unfaithful, then it will probably take a lot longer to release. But this is a starting point to be in touch with your feelings. The answers for this scenario could be – Yes, I can let go of this painful feeling but not until I get answers and find a new place to live.

The Sedona Method isn't about denying feelings. It's about awareness and attention.

Flower Essences, Bach Flowers Remedies, Even for Pets

Flower essences are tinctures made from the flowering part of a plant. Different flowers uniquely address a particular emotional and mental aspect of wellness. Flower essences can be used by adults, children, or pets. They're non-habit forming and can be used alongside other medicines. A popular flower essence company is Bach Flower Essences created by Edward Bach, an English physician and homeopath, in the 1930s.

Bach remedies come in little bottles with a dropper to be added to a drink. There are 38 remedies derived from different flowers, trees, and plants. Each remedy helps to alleviate a particular issue or emotional problem.

Examples of remedies:

Use Elm if you're overwhelmed by responsibility. This feeling can be frustration, exhaustion, or anxiety.

Use Impatiens if you're snapping at everyone and losing your patience quickly.

For children, Holly is helpful with anger issues, including sibling rivalry, and inability to accept a new baby in the family.

Mimulus is good for kids with nameable fears and phobias like the dark, dogs, or bugs.

If you're feeling a multitude of emotions, seven essences can be mixed at a time.

A premade combination remedy is available called Rescue Remedy which is appropriate for all urgencies and emergencies. It's made with Cherry Plum, Star of Bethlehem, Impatiens, Clematis, and Rock Rose. It can help with any stressful moment from going to the doctor, having an argument, or after an accident.

Flower essences work for pets. A remedy or a mix of remedies can help with separation anxiety (when the dog is destructive or whining), nervousness from fireworks, or incessant barking. Drops can go into drinking water or applied topically.

Need help deciding which to try? There's a plethora of books and websites that can help. There are also trained practitioners whom you can consult.

The Different Kinds of Therapists

When you look at the list of therapists in your health insurance booklet it doesn't indicate what kind of training these professionals have had or what kind of approach and methods they will use. Just as there are various massage therapy techniques (Swedish, Thai, mayofacial release) there are different methods of mental health therapy. Before you decide on a therapist, you can inquire about their training, the methods they use, and what their therapeutic approach is. A few of the talking therapies are: client-centered, existential, gestalt, narrative, Aldlerian, and CBT (cognitive behavioral therapy). A few alternatives to traditional talking therapy are art therapy, expressive art therapy (also known as creative arts therapy), biofeedback, music therapy, dance therapy, drama therapy, sandtray therapy, and play therapy.

The magazine *Psychology Today* has a listing on their website that explains the different therapeutic methods. http://therapists.psychologytoday.com/rms/content/therapy_meth ods.html

Expressive Arts Therapies Explained

Expressive arts therapies include art therapy, music therapy, dance therapy, drama therapy, writing therapy, play therapy, and sandtray therapy. It's also known as creative arts therapy.

Usually an expressive arts therapist has been trained in all these therapies but not to the same degree as someone who focuses on one modality. One expressive arts therapist may run groups in collage and group drumming due to the classes she has taken and the art forms she gravitates towards. Another expressive arts therapist might feel more comfortable working with drama and movement. But neither of these therapists would call themselves an art therapist or a music therapist per se, because those folks have more training and experience in that specific modality. For instance, music therapists need to be versed in piano, guitar, and voice. There are also board certifications to consider as well for each modality.

Now that the title has been explained, what does an expressive arts therapist do? That answer can literally fill a whole other book. But in a nutshell, they use the creative process with their clients in some way, shape, or form. Examples of a session include: group drumming with teens in jails to enhance team work and relive stress; drama therapy with an adult to address a childhood trauma and release the pain; painting with a child who lost a parent to process the grief and loss. The examples could go on and on.

Now what about expressive arts *facilitators*? These folks also use the creative process with their clients but not as therapy, not in a therapy setting, typically not with a diagnosed population, and usually not accepting payment from insurance companies. Expressive arts facilitators work with the general public out of their own studio spaces or in a variety of workshop settings. Some facilitators work in nursing homes, schools, hospitals, and with survivors of domestic abuse, and at schools. The Global Network of Expressive Arts Facilitators[28] is a good place to get more information about expressive arts facilitation and to find a facilitator near you. It's also a great resource if you need a multimodal workshop or retreat. For example, one facilitator can run a session on intuitive painting, another can run a session on somatic movement, and another could run a session on creating a vision board.

Now, what about expressive arts *coaching*? Expressive arts coaches are usually life coaches who use the expressive arts to help their clients.

---

[28] www.ExpressiveArtsFacilitators.com

Check Out the DSM

The DSM is the *Diagnostic and Statistical Manual of Mental Disorders* and it's used by therapists, clinicians, social workers, and psychologists to help diagnose their clients. Once a diagnosis is made, clients find relief by giving their issue a name. Thus treatment can begin and one can find support and support groups.

A therapist gets paid by an insurance company after she submits your diagnosis. You are entitled to ask what diagnosis she's assigned, if you wish. If having a diagnosis reported to your insurance company is a concern, you have the option to pay out of pocket. This can be discussed with your mental health provider *prior* to your first session.

The DSM is available at the library as a reference and to educate yourself. The book is divided into sections, such as mood, anxiety, sleep, gender, and childhood.

Walking the Labyrinths

Labyrinths are circular designs to be walked through as a kind of moving meditation. You walk to the center of it and then back out, repeating the process as many times as desired. Labyrinth formations are usually constructed outdoors and typically made of grass and stones. Many labyrinths are located in tranquil settings; strolling around one is often like a mini retreat. Brick labyrinths can be found in cities. My son and I recently walked an indoor labyrinth which was a very large canvas sheet. There are also small tabletop ones that you "walk" with your fingers.

Lea Goode-Harris, PhD, designer of labyrinths and sacred places and manages the Santa Rosa Labyrinth Foundation says that *"walking the labyrinth is an opportunity to let go of the past and come into the present moment of mind, heart, and feet connecting with the path beneath. The labyrinth is a place to find stillness, and a space to listen to your innermost thoughts. The goal of reaching the center is but a part of the journey. It is in staying present with every step of the path, both inward and outward, that meaningful truths are revealed. Within the twists and turns there is room to explore joy and sorrow, internal and external experiences, and to integrate the complexities of the times we live in."*

To find a labyrinth near you, go to www.labyrinthlocator.com. Also, the Labyrinth Society is coordinating future World Labyrinth Days, which are May 5, 2012 and May 4, 2013.

Brainwave Entrainment

Do you remember in high school learning about the two pendulum clocks that were moving out of sync but within a matter of time, they became in sync? Dutch physicist and mathematician Christiaan Huygens discovered this by accident. He invented the pendulum clock and noticed that his clocks would all sway in unison. Even after he misaligned them, they would all eventually swing in unison again. The reason behind this is due to entrainment, which is basically following the leader.

> *If you have two vibrating objects with the same natural frequency or corresponding harmonic, they will both have a forced vibration affect on each other. This process, given time, normally leads to a condition where both objects automatically synchronize. Once complete synchronization has occurred both oscillators are able to vibrate with less energy.*[29]

Isn't it interesting that more energy is needed and used when out of sync but when in sync, less energy is required? Now that's a metaphor for life!

When I was in graduate school, I took a drum facilitation class

---

[29] http://www.sound-physics.com/Sound/Entrainment/

and learned about entrainment as well. When people are making individual music on their hand drum or with a percussive instrument, within time, the group will come together and make a group song following the lead beat.

Brainwave entrainment follows the same logic. Brainwaves are electrical activity in the brain. When the brain is exposed to a certain frequency, your brainwaves will follow that frequency, thus you have brainwave entrainment.

> BETA waves are quick waves of 13 to 30 times per second (Hz). Beta brainwave patterns are generated naturally when we are awake and alert.

> ALPHA waves exist between 8 and 12 Hz. Alpha waves usually occur during rest (i.e. when the eyes are closed), intellectual relaxation, deep relaxation, meditation or when quieting the mind. Alpha waves are the desired result of experienced meditators.

> THETA waves exist between 4 and 7 Hz. This is commonly referred to as the dream or "twilight" state. Theta is associated with learning, memory, REM sleep and dreaming.[30]

---

[30] http://www.themorrymethod.com

If your brain is exposed to a sound with a lower frequency, such as 8 to 12 Hz like during Alpha waves, you'll feel calmer. Special audio recordings can change the state of brainwaves. There is research stating that brainwave entrainment can help with these issues: anxiety, athletic performance, stress reduction, attention (including ADD and ADHD), headaches/migraines, motivation, sleep and insomnia.

Purge!

Letting go of physical stuff can help with your mental and emotional health. It's cleansing to toss, recycle, sell, or donate to a charity your unused things and mementos that no longer bring you joy or that you no longer use. Releasing the clutter may allow more to flow in because the stagnate energy of your old stuff will be gone.

Have you ever watched a television show about cleaning out clutter? I appreciate when the tv show host discusses the psychological connections with the clutter. Guilt and fear are usually the root causes of holding onto stuff. Letting go of items passed down through generations or received as gifts triggers guilt. Guilt also surfaces when getting rid of items purchased but never used. Hard earned money was spent or credit cards were used to acquire the items so it seems ridiculous to get rid of them. These folks should give themselves a break, even forgive themselves, and be more aware of future purchases. Fear gets triggered when purging because people's stuff act as a security blanket. Scared thoughts run amok like "What if I need it one day?" and "Since I probably won't get any more, I have to hold on to everything."

A television show episode highlighted a couple's lovely furnished guest room, full of unused stuff from floor to ceiling covering the bed. Whenever the homeowner's elderly mother visited she had to sleep on the uncomfortable sofa in the cold, unwelcoming, unfinished basement. The show's host explained that this arrangement can be metaphorically translated to the homeowner "loving" her unused stuff more than her elderly mother's comfort. The homeowner had a revelation and then broke down crying. She was so unaware of how she allowed her stuff to control her. During the rest of the show the homeowner cleaned and cleared with joy and repeated, "I don't even know why I have this."

Remember this phrase when purging and decluttering - If it isn't a *Hell Yes!*, then it's a *Hell No!*. There are no *Hell Maybes*. Should I donate this piece of exercise equipment I haven't used in years? *Hell Yes!* Should I get rid of the concert shirt I've had since college? *Hell No!* I smile every time I look at it even though I don't wear it. It was such a fun night and it brings me joy.

ABOUT THE AUTHOR

Gabrielle Javier-Cerulli has a M.A. in Expressive Arts Therapy and has worked with all ages from children to seniors. After a variety of work as a clinician, she wished to be leave the world of diagnosing and insurance limitations. Instead she wanted to bring the expressive arts experience to the general public.

Thus, she opened her doors as The Expressive Arts Coach and offers workshops, sessions, and products which help people engage in the creative process so they may benefit from self-discovery and simply for the joy of exercising their Creative Self!

www.TheExpressiveArtsCoach.com

You can download 3 creativity exercises that you can do right now from this website!

She has also written an ebook, *Create Your Vision Board at Home: Learn to clarify your needs, desires, and goals using your creativity* so people can complete this personal project in the comfort of their homes and not have to travel to a workshop. It comes with over 150 reflection questions to help you make the most honest vision board for you.

Gabrielle believes in the power and benefits of the expressive arts so deeply that she founded the Global Network of Expressive Arts Facilitators where a wide variety of professionals using the creative process with their clients come together as an online community. GNEAF is also a place where the general public can find a facilitator and workshops near them and learn more about the field.

www.ExpressiveArtsFacilitators.com

At this website, you can sign up for the e-newsletter and weekly inspirational quotes!

She is also an abstract painter, enjoys hikes, and her current favorite color is vermilion orange.

You know you are no ordinary woman but you need help in unveiling your true self.

Change Your Life with the

No Ordinary Woman Toolkit

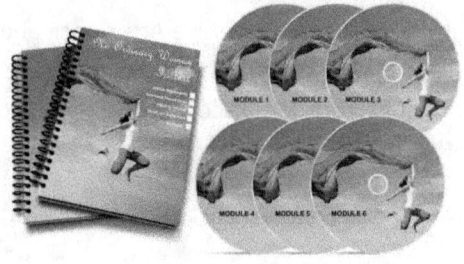

✓Engage in Much Needed Self-Care

✓Understand Yourself Better

✓Exercise Your Creative Self

✓Raise Your Vibration

through 6 modules of audio recordings and how-to videos

For more info, go to
www.NoOrdinaryWoman.net
Any questions? Email at NOWnordinarywoman@gmail.com

www.ingramcontent.com/pod-product-compliance
Lightning Source LLC
Chambersburg PA
CBHW070137290526
45789CB00002B/519